NIRVANA BLUES

A NOVEL BY
CHRIS CORBETT

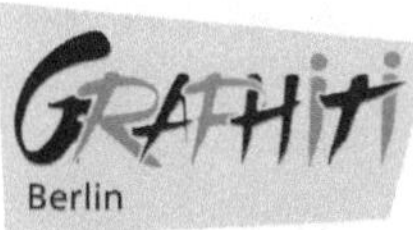

GRAFFITI
Berlin

Graphiti Publishing
Dieffenbachstrasse 78, Berlin, Germany 10967

ISBN 978-3-945383-92-6

Grateful acknowledgement is made to the following for permission
to reprint previously published material:

Take My Love
Lyrics: M. Lanning, T. Hilton, J. Strauss
Used by permission of the artists.

Silence Speaks
By: Baba Hari Das
Used by permission of the Sri Rama Foundation.

MAIA

Illusion works impenetrable,
Weaving webs innumerable;
Her gay pictures never fail,
Crowd each other, veil on veil;
Charmer who will be believed
By man who thirsts to be deceived.

Emerson

1

JOURNEY TO THE EAST

Stephan Collins was trying to look brave in front of a friendly crowd of Indian men who were gently pushing each other to get a better view of what was going on in the telephone cabin he was guarding. Stephan was on duty in a corner of the broad stone platform behind the Rishikesh train station, an ancient building that hadn't changed since the 1930s with arched doorways, clay tiled roof and walls painted a faded tan color like in a sepia photograph. The station was the end of the line where the steep Himalayan foothills covered with dense forest made laying further tracks impossible.

It was late in the afternoon of a cloudless day that let the azure sky show its glory and the temperature had dropped to a mild, lazy heat. The platform was deserted after the second of the two daily trains to Hardwar had left an hour earlier but a small group of local people had gradually accumulated, attracted by the sight of two young foreigners engaged in something unusual and possibly illegal. Foreign travelers were always a minor event in the remote mountain town even after the Beatles had visited with their entourage eight years earlier in 1968 and triggered a wave of youths going on the hippie trail. But Stephan's worn polo shirt and ancient chinos made him appear more serious and academic than the usual peace-and-love types wearing long kurta shirts and beads.

Stephan was leaning against the doorframe of the cabin with weathered red paint looking like it belonged on a street corner in London. He was trying to provide space for his friend James Montage and to let some air in to dispel the smell of old urine and centuries' worth of grime. The cabin was like a sauna after the two of them had been squeezed inside for half an hour.

James was juggling the phone handset that he'd attached to a homemade electronic device, a black metal box the size of two decks of playing cards with a telephone keypad on the top and a cable on the end. This was linked to the device's flat, cup-shaped connector clamped over the mouthpiece of the ancient phone. Brushing his matted, long dark hair out of his narrow face with the back of his hand, James started pushing buttons that created audible tones ranging from sharp beeps to a high-frequency screeching sound.

"This phone must be left over from the British Raj. I can't even get a decent dial tone to hack from. And I sure as hell ain't going to pay a zillion rupees to call California," James said.

"Maybe you should just trust Grok. He's not going to run the business into the ground."

"With my luck, he's probably goofing around designing what he thinks is the next cool thing. And I'm sure my marketing guy's off getting high somewhere."

"When you reached him from Delhi it was business as

usual." Stephan tugged at the neck of his damp shirt in an attempt to cool off.

"That's what worries me. Grok sounds okay but I don't think he's happy in our new offices."

Stephan reminded him that there was also some adult supervision in the form of a new investor who was mentoring the young team that comprised James's company as they tried to invent the future. He teased James saying that the real purpose of calling was to see if his girlfriend still remembered him, which he denied. When they had been able to get through to the office from a more modern phone in Delhi the seeming lack of enthusiasm from the lady James had been dating disheartened him. Stephan assured James that their friend Greg was surely taking care of her, as his passion for women was only second to his love of cars. James gave a stare in reply that said the joke was over but then quickly broke into a smile and said Buddha's last temptation before reaching enlightenment was a gorgeous courtesan so perhaps he should also let go.

"Does this mean we can get on with our search for enlightenment?" Stephan said.

"To nirvana," James said, raising his hand in a salute with the device in his fist.

After four weeks of rambling around northern India, the two suburban yogis had ended up based at a backpacker hotel overlooking the sacred Ganges. Stephan had just left university where he had been studying journalism and was doing research for a novel based on the ancient warrior king Rama, modernizing the East Asian epic tale of honor, bravery and wise actions. He thought the story had timely themes illustrated by the various plots and sub-plots of family dynasties with jealous stepmothers, evil kings kidnapping beautiful princesses, loyal servants and inspired underdogs battling demons for the virtuous young prince Rama. Stephan would set the story in twentieth-century America to make it more digestible for a broader audience and illustrate the values he had discovered in his studies of comparative religions. Writing stories for a newspaper would certainly have been interesting but he first wanted to try his hand at a novel before jumping into a newsroom. He saw it as his contribution to making the world a better place after the idealism he had seen around him as a teenager faded out. James, having also been seriously interested in Eastern philosophy for some years, had taken a much-needed break from his young electronics company soon to enter a more serious phase of development. If he wanted to make this journey, it was now or never. And while he was inclined to meditation and yoga he wasn't sure how those studies were harmonious with driving a commercial endeavor as some of the teachings equated pursuing commerce with ego and greed. James had been known as a mad monk for his endless philosophizing in a liberal arts college that provided a creative environment of freethinking and drugs. It hadn't provided what he was yearning for so he dropped out. While gathering money for his eventual quest for truth he had a renewed interest in the newly developing area of microelectronics that was slowly taking hold of the sleepy valley of apricot trees and aerospace companies south of San Francisco that he called home. James had a sense there was a way to benefit humanity through new tools that could extend human capabilities and connect people.

A few weeks earlier they'd conducted a search amongst the many teachers, sadhus and saints at the Kumbh Mela festival, looking for anyone with authentic wisdom. This was the largest gathering of humans on the planet where 15 million devout Hindus came together every dozen years in one of four sacred cities along the holy Ganges to wash away their past karma. But their short visit at the festival was fruitless as was their subsequent explorations around Rishikesh that was renowned for its large concentration of yogis and saints. They had met a variety of teachers who chanted, read from scriptures and lectured on the brotherhood of man but none of them gave the feeling of having the ability to show the practical experience of what they were talking about.

Before they'd come to India, one teacher in particular had been the focus of their searching and the catalyst for their journey: Neem Karoli Baba. This enlightened master had been discovered in the late sixties by a Harvard psychology professor named Richard Alpert. The professor had become a yoga student as he could only explain with ancient Eastern philosophy the far out spaces he had entered using psychedelic drugs to explore new psychiatric healing approaches with his fellow researcher Timothy Leary. The yoga teacher had shown him the meditative way to 'be high' rather than the 'get high' process the professors had been practicing. Even though the teacher's wise words were widely dispersed in a bestseller Alpert wrote called *Be Here*

Now that became standard reading on college campuses in the early seventies, his whereabouts were kept hidden to protect his privacy with only obscure clues indicating his general location. Stephan and James had each read the book many times and finding this teacher who really 'knew' became their obsession.

The son of a restaurant owner in Rishikesh had befriended the pair after their daily visits for mango lassis, sharing with them reports from earlier seekers who had discovered the location of the teacher. They set off trekking up and down forested ridges in the Himalayan foothills and finally found their way to the remote temple where Neem Karoli spent most of his time. The compound of small, whitewashed buildings, some with conical spires, was perched on a steep ridge covered with pine trees. From his studies in college of holy texts and books like *Autobiography of a Yogi* that explained the path to enlightenment sparked by contact with saint-like wise men, James had imagined a mind-reading session and instant clarity from a blessing by the reclusive sparkly-eyed teacher. This would induce a deep blissful experience known as samadhi, just like the Harvard professor had experienced years earlier.

Both men were filled with trepidation; many seekers who had eventually found the place had been turned away because of their lack of respect or preparation. After all the weeks of hiking and searching they wanted to have a genuine encounter with someone who wasn't playing games. They felt they had paid their dues by carrying on with their quest in spite of all the built-in challenges such as a case of 'Delhi belly' in a land that didn't have toilet paper as a standard convenience. Stephan was sure he had drunk enough over-sweetened chai, been sufficiently bounced around with his intestinal problems on the back of rickety busses and had slept on enough hard, wooden train station benches to deserve some form of acknowledgement of his persistence. If there were further tests to challenge his seriousness, he couldn't imagine what they might be. While he wasn't as fixated as James on a hit of nirvana, Stephan had wanted to hear some authentic interpretations of Indian teaching stories to help him build his novel with a deeper dimension.

After announcing themselves at the temple entrance they were shocked to find the famous teacher had passed away a few months earlier. At the same time, they were also deeply saddened at the loss of the great teacher. With the news of Neem Karoli's passing they had to rethink their strategy and even a pilgrimage to the source of the holy Ganges seemed like a tourist jaunt rather than a quest for inner peace.

As the slate of objectives, concepts and expectations had been wiped clean, James and Stephan agreed that all that was left was to let the cosmos decide if anything would happen in their final weeks in India. They were both deeply disappointed at the missed chance and momentarily disoriented as to their next steps but agreed to keep on truckin' and set off for a small town by a mountain lake called Nainital. The green-hued lake was in the region of the Almora hills, a location full of temples and spectacular views of the Himalayas and was also one of the areas to pursue their Plan B, searching for an ageless avatar named Babaji, who had been seen on and off there since the 1800s. They could make themselves available if this other teacher wanted to announce himself and guide them as he had many other serious students who had eventually documented their encounters. Besides, further along the foothills was a valley that served as India's main marijuana growing region centered on a town called Manali where according to legend, Manu, the Indian Noah, landed with the first humans after a great flood to populate the planet. If no saints adopted them, some good herb and mellow vibes were an eventual consolation prize.

After looking in on some sacred sites, sleeping on temple floors and longing for fulfillment, they spent a few days by the lake in Manali enjoying the solitude. One morning they decided to head back to Hardwar for their eventual train back to Delhi and started on a different route that went further north along the base of the Himalayan range. The going was slow, as it was hot during the day and dusty, and James was a bit depressed mostly owing to the hangover that followed all the hashish he had smoked with some German backpackers the night before. Neither one of them held out much hope for finding some wisdom after all the useless encounters, but they set off on foot, hitch-hiking when they got too tired to walk.

Walking down a dirt cart track, Stephan, ever the positive thinking spokesman, tried to break through their funk. "I think we're almost ready."

"Ready for what, another round of the 'Curse of Calcutta'?" James quipped, hitching his heavy pack higher on his back. He had reluctantly given up his raw-foods diet when dysentery struck because he had ignored the warning of 'cook it, peel it or don't eat it'. He had now adapted to the local cuisine but was skinnier than ever. His weight loss was accentuated by his being taller than Stephan, while his slim build and dark features on a long face that was framed by shoulder-length hair made him look European. By contrast, Stephan's square face, stocky build and collegiate haircut were typical of a Mid-western farmer.

"Not exactly. That was part of the purification but if you're honest we're only a couple of tourists. If we were hungry for a real experience then we would find it."

"When the student is ready the teacher will appear," James said.

"Buddha," Stephan said like he was answering a game show quiz. "I don't think all these wise guys are just selling books and seminars, they want to see if you are really sincere or only taking in the sights," Stephan said as he carefully circumnavigated a pile of cow dung in the middle of the path.

"Sure, but until now all we've met are swamis who can run a handkerchief up their nose and pull it out their ass. And then there are all those dirty sadhus with matted hair, chillums and open hands for rupees. What are you going to learn from somebody who claims to have given up the material world by standing on one foot in the Ganges while rattling his begging bowl? We've got a week and a half left and all I can think of is a real mattress and a giant pizza with greasy cheese floating on a sea of pepperonis."

They grumbled their way another couple of miles along the dirt road separating fields of sugar cane, Stephan ever-watchful for stray cobras. Later, the two of them were sitting outside a small hut at the outskirts of a village, eating samosas and sipping chai, when a sadhu with a beard and hair piled in a cone, clothed in a worn-out dhoti and kurta, sat down a short distance away watching them. These wandering monks who renounced all material possessions to dedicate their life to search for God were a common sight, and by now the two Westerners understood to have spare coins for beggars and sadhus. Stephan went over and offered him some rupees, but the man didn't accept them. The sadhu reached into a shoulder bag and took out a small chalkboard. He wrote some block letters in English:

What is the aim of your wandering?

Stephan called James over and they sat in front of the man both totally surprised to see a native in the middle of nowhere, an area of only sugar cane fields and small villages out of the Stone Age, writing in English.

"We're looking for the truth," Stephan said studying the man.

The sadhu wiped the board with a rag and wrote: No truth in America?

James answered, "America's too materialistic. India is where the truth is."

No God in America?

James and Stephan looked at each other and couldn't think of an answer. This dialogue went on for another half hour, and each time Stephan and James would rationalize an answer, a clear, simple reply would stop them in their tracks. The sadhu instructed them to stay there that night. They figured there were no pressing engagements so decided to accept his suggestion and besides, this sadhu had a special way of addressing their questions they hadn't encountered before. Stephan had copied down the words in his notebook like a good journalist and he and James talked about them over dinner.

The next morning, when they climbed out of their sleeping bags, the sadhu was sitting under a nearby neem tree. While they had a breakfast of yogurt, chapatis and some curry the local Indians had prepared for them as a courtesy, the sadhu started again with the conversation where they sat against a small hut that was the local shop.

Have you seen God?

James leaned over and whispered to Stephan, "I once smoked five joints and drank a bottle of vodka and had a mystical experience."

Where love comes from?

Have you peace?

"Of course we have peace, what do you mean?" Stephan asked.

Why did you leave America?

"We wanted to see if there were any real teachers who could show us an authentic experience because this land is known for that tradition. So far it looks like only beggars and merchants selling their solutions," James said.

Is peace God?

"Of course, and God is love, and love is God," Stephan said.

Then why did you leave America? Peace is there as much as here.

The two were momentarily speechless. Once in a while he would write:

Have you seen the light of God?

"Of course, hasn't everyone?" James answered the question with his own question.

Every morning the two travelers would wake up, get their sleeping bags rolled up, and the sadhu would start another dialogue.

Why did America kill Kennedy? Why did America make bombs? Why did people kill Jesus Christ? Why did people kill Rama, Krishna?

And in-between all these questions he would write:

The mind is the tool of the devil.

The sadhu was genuinely happy and sometimes they would play like children, laughing and rolling in the dirt. And throughout their discussions the silent baba emanated a feeling of presence and clarity that made it impossible for Stephan and James to leave him. It was like the permanence and stability of the Rock of Gibraltar combined with the depth and transparency of the deepest ocean. It became slowly clear to the two students that this guy Knew.

One day the silent baba took them for a walk that started out at sunrise and went on until sundown. Even though he had never spoken to them and only communicated by writing, on this day he didn't write a single word. As they walked amongst the fields and scattered forests under a relentless sun, he would point with his cane at everything. He would aim the stick at a plant in the field, and the two friends would look at it. While walking, he would point to a bird, the sky, flowers, barbed wire fences, sugar cane, insects, and many different things.

They walked all day without eating or stopping, and finally at sunset they rested on a small hill, to watch the sun go down over a forested plateau. The baba slowly moved his cane in a big circle and, as he made this motion, he held up a single finger to indicate the number 'one'. It was a moment of unexpected clarity and at that instant Stephan felt connected to every atom in existence, understanding all things were part of one universal energy. James followed the lesson intellectually and nodded slowly in agreement with the theory and technique of delivery. While the simplicity touched him, the help he was looking for to understand the material world and how to live in it and not be attached to its temporary pleasures was still unanswered. It was silent with only the buzz of insects and distant chatter of birds and the two young men gradually felt they were in a deep well of silence and all knowing that seemed to stretch beyond forever. Eventually Stephan slowly turned and looked at James and could see he had also been moved.

Stephan said in a soft voice that what they had been learning with the baba was clear – it didn't matter where you lived, peace was wherever you were, so going back to America wasn't an ending. Even though their external journey was over for now, they had a stronger sense that truth existed and if they persisted, somehow they would find it.

After returning to the village they said their farewells to the baba and exchanged hugs. The baba gave them the name of an ashram where he was a frequent guest in the event they wanted to find him again.

Two days later back in Hardwar, James and Stephan crossed a near empty footbridge to a small beach along the river where some bamboo-framed food and trinket stands were located. It was their last day in the holy city known as the Gateway to the Gods because of its location where the Ganges left the mountains and entered the plains, and the next morning it was back to Delhi and onto America. Their cheap tickets had a fixed departure date, and in spite of it being an unbelievably inexpensive country, their meager amount of money was almost gone. At one of the stands they each bought round boats the size and shape of half a grapefruit, fashioned from broad shiny green leaves with a center of golden flowers that looked like marigolds. There was a small candle in the middle of the blossoms, and the local tradition said that if your boat would make it out of sight down the river without sinking, your prayers would be answered. They went to the edge of the Ganges to launch them.

Nearby, a small group of Hindu devotees were singing Arati and swinging candles in the dusk before a little shrine built out of rocks on the riverbank with a picture of a reclining Shiva, the patron saint of yogis and sadhus. The two young men walked down to a sandy area by the water and squatted down and lit the candles. Stephan set his boat on the edge of the fast-flowing river, giving a small push, so the lit-up ship of dreams would catch the current. James watched for a second and gently dropped his boat into the swirling water and observed it getting pulled along, gradually picking up speed.

The blue-green Himalayan water chattered at their feet

in a timeless language as the boats swirled and dipped in the animated water. The two friends watched intently, fearing the vessels would capsize as the small waves in the river were rapidly lifting and dropping them. Soon the boats were drawn into the main current dancing along the ripples with their lit candles periodically winking with assurance at the two friends. Stephan and James looked at each other and shared an easy smile. James had been reflecting on how he could keep his aspiration for inner fulfillment alive while diving deep into the business world of deal making and driving for success. Stephan's wish was simpler, making a heartfelt vow to the silent baba to share his words so others could also find a place of peace in their heart. The small floating prayers were buffeted by the waves and bounced along in the flowing water slowly rounding the bend out of sight.

They knew they needed to return to their rented rooms before dark partly because of the threat of wild, nocturnal animals. They clambered over some rocks and followed a dusty path through a thicket of reeds emerging at the edge of an expanse of rice paddies with the vibrant green muted in the falling light. The footpath led around the edge of the field to a cart trail they followed into the forest carefully avoiding the sides where human waste lay in piles from where the nearby villagers routinely relieved themselves. A couple of men wearing only shorts and turbans passed them carrying bundles slung over their shoulder and greeted them with the traditional 'Ram, Ram' to wish 'God be with you'. It was still warm so the forest air was thick with a mix of exotic scents and Stephan was sure he caught a whiff of patchouli reminding him of every hippie he had ever met. The trail eventually left the cover of the trees and widened at a small collection of mud and brick huts with a couple of shops built on either side of the rutted dirt track. Wild forest stretched in all directions beyond the village, and as Stephan and James approached the settlement they dodged feral dogs on the prowl that paused briefly to sniff them suspiciously.

A local tour guide named Chat Rap Prat who had been helping with travel arrangements called to the two of them from an open-air food stand. They flopped down on simple folding chairs next to the young man who was wearing a threadbare dress shirt, worn-out polyester slacks and flip-flops that looked ready to fall apart at any moment. Chat Rap sat at a small rickety wooden table that was one of several on a cement patio enclosed by a low, whitewashed brick wall. After exchanging greetings and providing a short update on their river ceremony, James and Stephan ordered tea from a polite young waiter who was bustling around. It was an effort for the two Americans to speak with Chat Rap as he was unusually quiet, staring vacantly into the distant Sal trees.

The guests at the other tables weren't eating so the gas grill behind a plaster wall that defined the kitchen area was quiet except for the chef cooking their chai, stirring an aluminum pot frothy to the brim with boiling milk and spices. The tantalizing smell of ginger and cardamom made James and Stephan slowly think about food. They watched the intermittent flow of people wandering by, chatting excitedly on their way to the center of the village, and an occasional stray mongrel dog would pause for a moment and sniff expectantly hoping for a few morsels of food. The villagers at the neighboring tables were talking excitedly with exaggerated gestures punctuating their highly animated conversations. There were passionate arguments and angry shouting amongst the other guests as they argued back and forth intensely in local dialect. The tea was served and after paying and thanking the waiter James asked Chat Rap what was going on.

Chat Rap sighed deeply before replying. "I think it is best that we find you accommodation in another village."

"What's the problem? I don't mind sleeping on a charpoy – ropes for a mattress sure look weird but it's better than the benches in a train station," James said taking a sip from his tea.

"The village elders are reviewing the case of a young lady who has been accused of adultery. And as is the custom she will have to walk through a fire unscathed to prove her fidelity." Chat Rap was still staring at the distant fir trees as he spoke.

"What? I thought that practice had stopped long ago," Stephan said.

"Ah – yes. This is an ancient custom from the time of Rama thousands of years ago. Now it's a common way the husband can be rid of his wife," Chat Rap said in his sing-song voice as his head bobbed slowly from side to side.

"What do you mean rid of her?" James said. He put his cup down and was staring intently at Chat Rap.

"In India women are considered possessions that don't bring much to a marriage which is why her family must pay a dowry to make things equal. If further requests for money aren't met the husband can make a false accusation and replace his wife with one whose family has more money."

"And what about love – doesn't that count for anything?" Stephan said.

"In our society marriages are arranged to the best advantage of both families. Love will come later," Chat Rap said.

"Is the woman sent home when they divorce?" James said.

"If she is lucky. Usually there is a deadly accident like a kitchen fire. In this test today if the wife does not emerge from the flames without burns the punishment is to be devoured publicly by dogs." There was a moment of silence as Chat Rap looked at the two Americans with an expression of shame.

"You've got to be kidding," Stephan said. "That's totally barbaric."

"You can forget about writing your peace-and-love Rama story now," James said finishing his tea with a flourish.

"This can't be supported by the *Vedas*. Those holy books are the basis for the Hindu religion and talk about the value of life," Stephan said to Chat Rap.

"Like in all religions the rules get interpreted by priests to suit their own views," Chat Rap said holding his hands up in a gesture of surrender.

"If it ain't changed in thousands of years it's not going to change anytime soon," James said. "So much for a country with a culture of spirituality." Stephan held the clay teacup tightly in his hands and stared into the depths. "It doesn't matter, we have to stop this from happening," James said looking at Chat Rap.

"Once the Pradhan has made his decree we cannot do anything. He is the final authority in the village," Chat Rap said.

"And the bride's family? Don't they have a say?" Stephan said looking up.

"They are usually very in debt from borrowing for the original dowry so they cannot pay to change the verdict or even begin to dream of money for a second dowry. So somehow it is the best for them also." Chat Rap recited the words like he was reading poetry.

"Let's get the police," James said pushing back from the table.

"The closest police station is ten miles away and the two policemen are never there because of the many villages in their territory."

"Then I'm going to talk to this mayor guy," James said.

"He is as corrupt as any politician and has most certainly received a bribe to make a ruling against the bride," Chat Rap said with a tone of futility.

"This is so fucked-up. I can't believe I'm hearing this," James said. "We have some dollars, I'll pay off this thug or the groom – I don't care."

"Your money will not help. We lead a life based on divine order to be true to our dharma, accepting what the universe provides. This you cannot change."

"I don't care, I'm going to put a stop to this," James said.

"The whole village will be against you. This is their tradition."

"Bullshit!" James jumped up and quickly stepped over the low patio wall and jogged a few hundred meters around the buildings to a clearing where a six-foot tall pyramid of tree branches was stacked ready to be lit. A small crowd of men in sarongs and T-shirts and women in a rainbow of saris were standing around expectantly, chattering among themselves.

Stephan and Chat Rap caught up to James as he was looking around in the crowd for someone of authority to talk to. A couple of local men in sandals, linen pants and ancient dress shirts acting as police and brandishing long bamboo truncheons were positioned in front of a small one-story building with a flat roof that housed the local township office. A beat-up mud-colored Maruti jeep was parked askance by the corner. James charged towards the building but one of the men cut off his approach holding the bamboo club crosswise in both hands.

"You will leave now," the man said in strong British-accented English mixed with a Hindi twang. He pushed the club against James's chest, forcing him back. James stumbled but regained his footing and as he started to make a grab for the man Chat Rap and Stephan each caught an arm and pulled him away. James resisted at first but resigned himself to the retreat as the second guard approached menacingly also with his lathi ready to strike.

As the three interlopers were herded away from the village center the crowd got louder. James and Stephan turned to see what was going on and the two policemen also paused to look back, more interested to observe the spectacle than escort the foreigners.

An old man lit the fire and the tangled branches quickly ignited with a loud roar sending flames five feet in the air with a billowing spiral of white smoke. As if on cue, the two families came out of the building wearing traditional clothing. One of the older women in a red sari and severe face led the way. An attractive girl in her late teens with long black hair pulled back in a braid followed in a bright yellow sari sobbing hysterically. Her parents accompanied her on either side with distraught looks, the mother wailing as the girl gripped her parents' arms for support. Behind the family the father-in-law and husband followed with serious expressions. The entourage paused a few yards away from the fire waiting for the signal from the Pradhan, a rotund balding man in a dark blue silk dhoti and kurta who was following the small group with an air of authority.

From where James and Stephan were standing the heat waves from the fire distorted their view, lending everything a dreamlike quality like watching the proceedings from behind a curtain of water. The wind shifted and the dense smoke blew towards them stinging their eyes. The two Westerners were spellbound, staring with disbelief while the tableau unfolded. James kept looking over at the family, debating whether he should try and intervene, tensing his body to make a dash towards the group but the presence of the two guards kept him from action and he resigned himself to watching. Stephan felt like he had been transported back in time two thousand years and dropped into one of the last scenes in the Ramayana story where Rama's wife had to undergo the same test after she was rescued from the evil king to prove she hadn't slept with him. Rama's wife Sita was a goddess and had easily survived the ordeal but looking at the innocent bride Stephan knew the outcome wouldn't be a cause for celebration. He also felt compelled to shout out and disrupt the ceremony but a sense of helplessness kept him silent. The young girl was now wiping the tears off her cheeks while she regained her composure and stopped crying to stand tall and proud. Her face soon went blank with a hardened look as if she had aged twenty years in the exchange of a breath. She stepped away from her parents and walked awkwardly towards the fire with mechanical marionette-like movements. The crowd had also become silent with only the sound of crackling, flaming wood accompanying the ceremony.

The girl reached the edge of the fire and the hem of her sari ignited as she stepped carefully into the burning branches. The mother started shrieking and her husband had to wrap his arms around her waist to keep her from running after their child while the rest of the family watched dispassionately. None of the villagers made a move to stop the girl as they jostled for a better view. Stephan again wanted to shout out a warning but he felt powerless, overwhelmed by what was unfolding. He started sobbing as the enormity of the event hit him.

The fire quickly spread up the sari engulfing the girl in a sheath of flames. She frantically tried to rid herself of the burning clothing with sweeping motions as panic took over. She was screaming now but didn't run from the fire. Her mother was hysterically shouting out Hindi phrases and wailing like a woman possessed, echoing her daughter's cries. As if hearing some inner command, the girl stopped her panicked movements and quieted herself, bringing her scorching hands together in prayer position in front of her chest as her hair ignited in a halo of intense heat, flaming like burning straw as she stumbled forward across the burning branches trying to cross the fire.

For James the horror of it was more than shocking, it called everything into question, the baba's teachings on compassion and his own belief in man's ability to evolve to a more knowing, benevolent stature – it all meant nothing if actions like this were allowed to take place. He cursed his helplessness in the situation and the Pradhan for allowing the ritual. Stephan was gasping for breath as he stood there frozen with disbelief, watching the nightmare as tears streamed down his face seeing selfish cruelty acted out in the name of God. The girl continued to burn, and at last she let out the most blood-curdling cry the two Americans had ever heard. On the edge of the crowd, a sadhu, wearing the traditional cover of ashes from a cremation ghat and holding a begging bowl made from the crown of a human skull to show deference to death had to avert his eyes from the sight.

One of the policemen prodded the three young men down the dirt street with his bamboo stick until the fire was out of sight behind the small buildings. They could hear a roar go up from the crowd and then they were out of earshot. As they walked slowly back towards the café a couple of small groups of yipping dogs passed them heading towards the fire. James kicked out at one of them in frustration.

"Forget it, James, this is India," Stephan said in a pent-up voice, putting his hand on James's shoulder as they shuffled along ahead of Chat Rap.

Chat Rap came alongside the two young men and spoke with a tone of resignation. "That girl's life ended the day her parents sold her. And today she was accepting her karma by performing the correct action to take her to a better place."

"I hope you're right," James said choking on the words. "Otherwise that poor child sacrificed her life for a handful of rupees."

2

THE MERRIEST OF PRANKSTERS

Greasy Greg swept a pile of safety glass fragments towards the tow truck that was blocking the inside southbound lane of the El Camino Real in a run-down section of Palo Alto. He watched the rounded glass chunks reflect rainbows and scattered light refractions as they tumbled, sounding like pebbles on a beach being tugged by a receding tide. The cars in the adjoining lane contributed to the illusion with an occasional swooshing sound. Each rhythmic push of the broom generated new color variations in a mosaic of winking suns tumbling and growling through a parallel universe.

It was early evening, not a lot of traffic, streetlights blinking on in the developing dusk and commuters easing their way around the accident scene without showing much interest. A crunched-up Plymouth Duster was securely winched high by its nose, sitting on its two back wheels like a dog patiently begging for a biscuit.

Greasy's sweeping was broken by a shout from the truck's cab. "Hey, space case, get it together. I got to get up to the city tonight!"

Greasy looked up and waved the driver over, not too

bothered by the man's tone of voice. Cool Breeze jumped out of the cab and stomped over with a cardboard box for the glass pieces. His halo of wild hair accentuated his outfit of heavy biker boots, grimy jeans and 49ers football team sweatshirt with no sleeves. He tossed the box on the ground. Greg's look matched his except the jeans were boot cut, covering black Converse sneakers while a beat-up denim work shirt gave him a just-out-of-prison look. His face had the openness of an Amish farmer complete with goatee, short tousled hair and mischievous eyes beaming through round, wire frame glasses.

"Let's get this wreck down to the yard so we can check out," Breeze said.

"No problem. I have to teach a yoga class in an hour."

"Yogurt? You still into that scene?"

"Yeah, it's how I keep flexible so I can work on motors. Besides, a little elevated focus once in a while never hurts."

"Sounds like what we were telling folks at the Acid Tests a couple years back: 'go beyond'."

"And now?" Greg asked while trying to calculate how many times Breeze had repeated this phrase in the last month, as he scooped up the field of shards. Maybe Breeze really had lived the life if he couldn't remember it anymore.

"The seeds have been sown, the genie's out of the bottle. There's a lot of heat now, but the party goes on."

"Be careful when you back up. This rig could jackknife and rip the bumper right off our precious wreck."

"Who's driving, you or me?" Breeze said.

"No question about it. You're the captain for all the right reasons. I just don't want to have any pay deducted for mangling some little old lady's Sunday special if you know what I mean."

"I should steer left?"

"Reading my mind. I can see why I'm just your co-pilot." After a last tug on the winch to make sure their load was secure, they jumped in the cab and headed south towards Sunnyvale.

"So, how you figure the party goes on?" Greg said. "When we were cruising with Kesey and Cassady we were just living easy and helping people find that cool place inside."

"Yeah, for sure. But the fucking media killed the scene by making it look so hip. Everyone for a thousand miles wanting to live the dream showed up. The real freaks had already moved to the country and the inspiration died out. You party with your local tribe nowadays, stay cool and keep from getting busted," Breeze said.

Greasy pulled a half-smoked joint out of the ashtray and lit it. "Sounds like you gave up. Should be taking the next step in your personal evolution."

"Fuck you. I'm just living. You get so hung up on trying to put some spiritual framework around your life. Forget it, just keep moving on and go with the flow."

"Sounds cool but you're not accepting responsibility for your life, drifting from one six-pack to the next with a dose of speed here and there and some Colombian buds to mellow out on. It's like you're living in the past when 'anything goes' was breaking new ground. There needs to be some meaning to the madness, not perpetuating it. There's a lot of potential to help bring in a new age of awareness."

"Nude age? Naked chicks – far out. Okay, wise guy, what do you suggest?" Breeze said grabbing the joint.

"The past is history and future's a mystery, so enjoy this sweet moment."

"And what about your contribution to paradise on earth – fixing up cars so they can make more pollution?"

"Just tuning the beasts to burn cleaner. My plan is to one day open a garage called Karmic Annex. People can do yoga waiting for their oil change."

"Groovy. I remember when your buddies came back from India and they were wearing those pajamas—" Breeze said.

"Dhoti and kurta."

"Whatever. What was it you all were on about then?"

"Remembrance. Be here now."

"Beer now? What do you want to remember here? Look at this shit." Breeze waved the smoking joint across the windscreen taking in the cheap strip malls, faded pastel apartment buildings and mid-sized Chevys symbolizing the growing suburban sprawl. A seed popped in the joint, arching over the seat like a descending meteorite, sending them both into animation to sweep it on the floor before it burned a hole anywhere.

"It's all an illusion," Greg replied, "whether you're in a cave in the Himalayas or Grand Central Station."

"Yeah, and I'm a fairy godmother. Poof, you're a pile of shit." The tow-truck veered slightly when Breeze waved his imaginary wand, causing the car they were towing to fishtail into the next lane, generating some angry honks. On the radio Linda Ronstadt was shouting 'you're no good' and the guitar solo was kicking in before the last chorus. Breeze passed the joint back and noticed something on the flat area of Greg's hand behind the thumb and index finger. There were two parallel arrows side by side drawn with a pen, pointing in opposite directions.

"What's that, you got a tattoo now?" Breeze asked pointing with his chin.

"Nah, just a little reminder to be aware of each breath. Every time I take a hit on a joint I get pointed to the present moment."

"Looks like a street sign for two-way traffic to me. Your karma ran over my dogma." Breeze downshifted as they approached the car lot. "Hold on!" Breeze swung the truck through a gate in a tall chain-link fence, bouncing the wreck against the right metal support post. The junkyard was filled with a variety of cars in varying stages of entering the next life as recycled tin cans, an accumulation of carcasses of spent lives. Everything from squashed Beetles to flat-footed Mustangs and expired Pintos were on display.

Pausing before getting out of the cab, Breeze gave a parting shot. "You get on with your way, and I'll get on with mine. But the best way is no way." He turned to look at Greg, his intense eyes framed by his scraggly beard and bushy hair, making the point of his existential, Buddhist view of existence.

Always having to get in the last word, Greg couldn't resist adding, "Peace, brother, we're on the same team. You got it, baby. Let me know if you hear of any good parties. Wouldn't mind meeting some more of those foxy ladies like at that Menlo Park gig."

Greg pulled his '48 Dodge milk truck onto the El Camino for the short drive to Lawrence Expressway. He edged over into the sporadic post-rush-hour traffic while nimbly shifting gears. There was no clutch, just a crash box requiring expert timing to shift at the right moment to avoid dropping the transmission through the floor. The truck lurched forward, creating a racket as two metal toolboxes slid across the empty storage area in the rear.

Greg exited the expressway on Homestead Road and headed east, passing the Cappaletti fruit-packing warehouse, boxed in by tall piles of three-foot high wooden crates. Greg grinned when he saw the hand-painted sign hanging on the wall that said 'Down With Technology, Up With Trees'. You really had to give these farmers credit for creating a protest mood to rally the public against the encroaching office developments. He found it amusing that establishment figures were co-opting the counterculture tactics that helped end the Vietnam War a year earlier. The lines were starting to blur between who was right and who was left.

The farmers had held a large demonstration the week before, trying to block the creation of one more technology campus on five acres of original farmland. In a scene reminiscent of the best Berkeley free speech riots, police on horses, backed up by tear gas, had finally been called in to break up the demonstration. Even a handful of hippies had sided with the farmers who normally would have rejected their support. Greg grinned when he thought of the sweet irony of the farmers including James's Eden Computers on their list of companies to target with actions, as his friend James was more like them than they imagined.

He remembered James bragging about how he spent time working on an apple orchard in Oregon communing with nature and expounding his idealistic dreams about helping the common man. But the farmers were unaware of his history. All they saw were people like James and the semi-conductor companies taking over their apricot drying sheds. Greg was imagining what the reaction would be when he asked James to autograph an anti-construction flyer with his picture on it. James's fledgling company was on the verge of a major expansion if everything went according to plan, which could only mean more office buildings or a technology center that made James the perfect poster child for the farmers' next campaign.

Greg passed a lone block of isolated prune orchards heavy with never-to-be-picked fruit, occupying the exact space a pre-fab house could fit. Greg pulled his truck over at the corner where Stephan was shooting baskets in the driveway of a suburban tract home with a stylized front designed to look like a barn. Half the houses in the development had a variety of this motif – tear down the farms and put up a Disney version. Stephan tossed the ball onto the lawn and went over to the truck.

Greg greeted him as he climbed into the cab and slid across the bench seat. "Hey, buddy," and gave him the soul shake, interlocking thumbs like ghetto brothers. "Ready to teach these old ladies how to bend themselves into a pretzel?" Greg asked. He put the truck in gear and headed down the quiet streets of the subdivision.

"Sure. Could use a little stretching myself. The old man's cranking up the pressure again for me to figure out what to do." Stephan's father thought a university degree in journalism meant Stephan should get into teaching or work at a newspaper. He'd been telling Stephan he was no longer legally responsible to support him. Said to figure out what career to pursue or else go back to school and get a real degree in something practical like engineering. And to complicate matters, he didn't consider writing a legitimate profession.

"I know what you mean; I got the same heat on the home front."

Greasy's dad had suggested they both become consultants to the big corporations that were sprouting up in the valley like weeds in an unkempt garden. He was convinced they could use their understanding of human nature combined with a self-confident, people-centered outlook to build flowcharts and realign company processes. They could use their natural communication skills and enlightened thinking to help employees embrace change via endless meetings and scrawls on flip charts all the while making a pile of money.

Their calm clarity could soothe and assure hassled executives while their out-of-the box thinking provided innovative solutions to age-old problems like 'we always did it this way so we will continue to do it this way'. The advice fell on mostly deaf ears even though it resonated more with Stephan whose university-learned discipline made him the more structured of the two while Greg's freethinking outlook provided the creative balance. And it was ultimately this more bohemian attitude that won out and made them reluctant to commit to the necessary classes. They maintained the pretense of an agreement to keep the old man off their back while they mooched beers and tuna sandwiches from the family kitchen. The idea of suits and college courses didn't appeal to the spiritual nomads going for the heart of the matter.

"At least you went to mechanics school and got a degree," Stephan said bracing himself on the dashboard while Greg navigated a corner.

"Was no big deal – would have rather gone with you and James to India."

Stephan explained how James wanted him to help put electronic gadgets together for his new company, but Stephan didn't think there was a future to it. After all, who's going to buy a computer? James had sold a bunch already but the customers are all propeller head hobbyists so how far can that go? Stephan's father had told him that IBM owned the computer market with seven or eight huge computers installed around the world and there wasn't much more interest or need than that. But James was acting like he was doing Stephan a favor to let him work at Eden Computers. Had even offered him a bunch of shares in the company to get him excited.

"I can't quite figure him out. One minute he's a sadhu wandering around India looking for the meaning of life and now he wants to build a big technology company and make a pile of money." They had crossed Homestead, heading back towards the El Camino and started to look for parking on one of the side streets lined with small apartment buildings.

"He's sure it will help the world. He's got a great argument as usual to justify his missionary attitude," Stephan said.

"With him it's more like the missionary position. I keep

telling him that he can't squeeze dollars through his third eye when he leaves his body."

The yoga class was being held in the living room of a 200-pound psychic lady named Isadora, who was the mother of one of Stephan's high-school friends. Isadora had met Greg at a spiritual fair and knew he and Stephan were like brothers due to their matching auras. Sure enough they hit it off from the moment she introduced them. Greg was about ten years older and looked at Stephan like a younger brother or protégé. To support the two budding yogis, the psychic opened up her living room and provided some of her past-life regression clients as the initial students. Both Greg and Stephan were highly qualified mail-order suburban yogis. They'd taken classes from a foundation established back in the 1920s by an Indian teacher named Yogananda who set up several retreats in Southern California. His autobiography was a manual on all things yoga including his stories of an ancient India complete with tiger wrestling saints and his lineage of teachers that included the deathless avatar Babaji whom Stephan and James had hoped to bump into in the Himalayas. Greasy had studied some of the philosophy and learned the postures to help him to twist around engine compartments, while Stephan checked out various scriptures and meditations, using hatha yoga to synchronize his breathing and stretch his muscles to enable long sitting sessions.

Greg had been a bright student in high school but the academic nature of the lessons bored him. When he wasn't playing the position of tight-end for the football team he spent as much time as he could cutting classes and fixing cars to pick up girls with. Then one day an older brother of a classmate had invited him to a party in Palo Alto that was taking place amongst several small houses on a small street named Perry Lane near the Stanford campus. The host was a former student named Ken Kesey who had recently achieved national notoriety with a bestseller called *One Flew Over the Cuckoo's Nest*. His gatherings played host to a highly talented group of artists, writers and musicians with all-night rap sessions discussing the meaning of life and future of society. Greg would be a fly on the wall absorbing all the creative conversations and joining in the festive activities that included cheap wine and marijuana. When the Perry Lane area was scheduled to be torn down Kesey bought a house in the redwood forests in the mountains behind Palo Alto and started a project to take a bus tour across the States with a crew of artists called the Merry Pranksters and share his brand of a free-thinking rolling celebration while recording the whole extravaganza. The film project was like a road movie and was called 'Search for the Cool Place' – an allegory for people finding and celebrating their own cool place inside that the Pranksters believed everyone had. Much to his disappointment, Greg's parents didn't permit him to go along as the mechanic on a later trip by the bus to Woodstock because he was still legally a minor.

During his frequent visits Greg bonded with a member of the Kesey clan called Neal Cassady and because of their mutual love of cars spent many hours in fast-talking sessions of spontaneously flowing ideas while fixing the various autos the Pranksters used to get around in. Cassady had been immortalized years earlier in the book *On the Road* and his beatnik wisdom and free-spirit lifestyle had naturally aligned him with Kesey and his crew who were too young to be beatniks and too old to be hippies. Greg's wiseguy non-stop monologues on any subject under the sun were already in place, and under the tutelage of Cassady it was like being in the finishing school for developing rapturous expressions to celebrate the moment called now. Cassady had already received the name 'Sir Speed Limit' for obvious reasons, so it was only natural Greg became known as 'Greasy Greg'. The Pranksters would claim that the two car lovers were the origin of the phrase 'motor mouth'.

The Prankster scene fragmented due to police harassment and the various members went their different ways. Greg went on to finish high school and then took off on his own adventures. One road trip had his thumb landing him in Iowa and a ride from a university professor that had turned into an extended stay of studying art for a month as a respected guest. Attending classes as a special visitor and holding discussions on art and aesthetics with students and teachers made Greg feel he could handle the academic world on his own terms. Later on, he had traveled on a huge flatbed truck with a makeshift house on the back that was home to fifteen to twenty hippies that bounced between music festivals in Colorado and Oregon.

Eventually in 1972 Greg landed at a communal house in Lake Tahoe where a lot of other people from the San Francisco area had drifted. There he used his powers of persuasion to convince some young sweet girls to use their bodies to earn rent money. Tahoe being Tahoe, drunken gamblers were easily hustled on the street for paid companionship and yet Greg confessed he always felt funky when the money changed hands. The Tahoe experience eventually got too weird, so in '74 Greg drifted back to Sunnyvale and eventually enrolled in an auto mechanics school in order to get certified in what he had been haphazardly practicing over the years. It was an attempt at permanence and being grounded after knocking on the gates of heaven and bouncing against the doors to hell.

The yoga class was a mix of old ladies and spiritual hangers-on who were gathered in the chintzy living room of Isadora's modest house. Hand-made doilies covered antique end tables, and the sofa had a huge quilt made out of crocheted squares with a subtle mix of mud brown and Pepto-Bismol pink. It had the harmonic vibrations of your favorite grandma's living room but the atmosphere soon changed.

The students followed the two yogis' every move, impressed at their flexibility. The class went through some breathing exercises to get their vital energy called prana activated, although most people hyperventilated, mistaking their dizzy lack of oxygen for a rush of primal life force. Then the two teachers took turns guiding the class through a series of Sun Salutations and different standing and seated stretching postures. They could even cross their legs while seated, a feat that few of the class members could imitate. An hour later, to finish the class, they all assumed the Corpse posture, lying flat on their back with arms and legs splayed. After Greg walked around checking everyone was in the right position, he also lay down and started with a visualization technique that led into a muscle-by-muscle guided relaxation starting with the feet and working up the body. The room got very quiet about halfway through and Stephan had to take over while the master yogi had relaxed himself into a state of deep sleep.

After a round of herb tea and accompanying spiritual rap with the happy students and some minor flirting with the young ladies in the class, the two yogis skipped their usual sauna in the spa room of an adult condo community that they could sneak into and went straight for their after-workout meal. Sitting in the back of the milk truck consuming their purifying diet of buttermilk and Dr. Bronner's all-in-one biological corn chips (with esoteric philosophy nobody understood covering the bag), Greg announced he was moving to a spiritual center over the hill, at the beach in Santa Cruz.

"I'm going to be their resident mechanic and part-time yoga teacher in exchange for room and board. I think its time you also made a move. I know a big house downtown where a bunch of students are staying and you can get a room. And the center I'm working for owns an organic bakery, so I'm sure they could offer you some work for your rent money."

"Sounds better than the last gig here working at the carwash. This valley is so conservative it's stifling my creativity."

"Forget that shit. You need to get on with your writing

free of your parents' pressure. Then we can look into opening a yoga studio of our own. I might even get my own garage together with a juice bar and classes to entertain the customers while they wait. Everything's possible."

3

VALLEY OF THE HEART'S DELIGHT

Stephan stood on a mountaintop above the Santa Clara Valley, between the half-buried boulders of an Ohlone Indian ceremonial site studying the colored cloud formations painted by the setting sun. A westerly wind animated the dry grass on the hillside in undulating waves. The cry of a red-tailed hawk circling a grove of redwoods that swayed in a rhythmic dance in a small canyon along the ridge broke his reverie. It was a fortuitous omen, a wake-up call from another time and place. Stephan imagined the spirit of an ancient medicine man was directing his attention to the present moment, and the view over Palo Alto, where the gentle curves of the bay contrasted the urban sprawl and hazy patches of orchards that certified the valley as The Prune Capital of the World.

Since they had returned from India a couple of months earlier, he and James had drifted apart, mostly because James was burying himself with a renewed passion in the development of his small company while Stephan worked on his writing in solitary intensity. James was stressed far more than usual because of making up for the lost time from his trip to India, as the investors who had supported his vision were demanding deliverables. This extra pressure was on top of his normal drive to beat the invisible clock ticking in his brain that said he had to race if he wanted to define the new industry standards and reach the masses first. On top of all the work pressure an upsetting incident that revived old horrors had made James seek out Stephan's company.

The development team had finished a major redesign of the motherboard so their machines would run faster and show animated graphics. The project leader hosted a barbecue and beer bash at his home in the Los Altos foothills after the many eighteen-hour days and working on weekends required to meet the deadline. James showed up halfway through the evening to show solidarity and to let off some steam before the relentless pace started again the next day. He had found some juice in the kitchen and was sunk in the cushions of a dilapidated sofa on the back porch of the wooden ranch-style house. He was deep in conversation with a girl wearing faded jeans and an old rock and roll T-shirt who he knew from school and was now a journalist at a local paper.

A grill had been set up on the lawn off to the right of the porch and a group of ever-hungry engineers had been circling it with paper plates waiting for the next round of burgers. One of them took a bottle of kerosene and squirted a jet on the coals, impatient with how long the new layer of charcoal was taking to light. Out of the corner of his eye James saw a flash of flame and heard some yells. Turning to see the source of the commotion he saw a longhaired young man in a flaming T-shirt frantically trying to smother the flames from where the kerosene had been blown back from the fire igniting his shirt and hair that had dangled too close. James watched transfixed, holding his breath in a state of shock, unable to race to the rescue or shout instructions as he was transported back to India for a second, hearing the young girl's screams of horror that were permanently etched into his brain. Another engineer had quickly pulled off his jeans jacket and flung it over the screaming man's head effectively smothering the flames and then he quickly rolled the fire victim to the ground to extinguish his clothing.

Everyone in the crowd was gasping, shocked by the scene, and James had a second wave of traumatic memories as the smell of singed hair drifted over making him relive the spectacle he had been trying to blot out of his memory. Seeing that the man was relatively unharmed beyond his singed hair and lightly scorched face James pushed himself up from the depths of the sofa and without saying goodbye to anyone quietly left the party. As head of the company he should have checked on the engineer personally but he couldn't handle the closeness of the memories. Ever since that night he had been having nightmares of trying to outrun forest fires as crackling flames chased him, and visions of firemen in asbestos suits walking into burning buildings to rescue screaming victims. Now whenever he saw smoke or bright flashes the horror was relived for an instant. The fire.

James was sitting a couple of yards from Stephan on a rough stone slab and was also taking in the panorama and Mount Diablo across the valley where thunderheads were building up, slowly moving in their direction.

James broke the silence. "Thanks for bringing me up here. I forgot what an amazing view this place has. But why the hell didn't we just drive here – that's Skyline Boulevard right below us." James didn't want to admit that the antibiotics for the unfriendly Indian microbes that had hitchhiked back home with him had been impacting his usual high energy level.

"I wanted our hike to be like the pilgrimage we did in India."

"It is pretty easy to get lost in this illusion, that's for sure," James said indicating the valley with a nod of his head. James went on to recount the incident with the fire and how he still couldn't free himself from the images of the burning girl. Stephan leaned against a large chunk of weathered granite and pulled a few round, spiky burrs off his socks and then idly watched the hawk riding thermals, floating west towards the coast over empty fields while James finished his story. Stephan listened respectfully and then shared an event that had the same effect of waking up old ghosts.

Stephan had been checking out classes at a human potential center in Oakland that offered encounter groups and Zen workshops and one of the instructors had given him a ride to the freeway on-ramp where he could hitchhike back to Santa Clara. Even in daylight it was unsafe to walk through the part of town between the house and the freeway, as it was the edge of the ghetto. During the drive they pulled up to a stop sign in a neighborhood of single-story tract homes that were on the verge of collapse. The front door of a run-down house next to where they were waiting burst open and a teenage girl with long hair wearing cut-off jeans and a halter-top came crashing out the front door, stumbled over the porch and fell in the dirt front yard as she attempted to run away. An older man with stubble and his belly half covered by a worn-out white T-shirt charged out after her cursing and waving a belt in one hand. As she scrambled to get away the man fell to his knees and grabbed an ankle, striking her on the back with the belt, shouting at her, calling her a whore. Dropping the belt, he grabbed an arm and twisted the girl around and slapping her face so hard she sprawled on her back. A car was honking behind Stephan, as his driver also engrossed by the scene hadn't noticed they were blocking the intersection, so they drove on without seeing what happened next. Stephan once again felt that sense of helplessness and injustice when witnessing a young girl being brutally mistreated.

There was a silence between the two friends as the wind rustled the tall grass and a distant car approached on the road below with a far-off buzzing sound. James stood up and started pacing the width of the flat area between the boulders.

Stephan spoke up. "Just when I thought I was starting to put that India scene behind me there it was again."

"Yeah, me too. With my crazy schedule it was almost a distant memory with only little flashbacks here and there."

"You know, it really messes with my head. I want to get on with my Rama story but sometimes I feel a hypocrite. I ask myself how I can talk about enlightened living when I did nothing to save an innocent girl's life."

"Man, I can say the same thing. But if either of us had tried to save the girl we'd be rotting away in an Indian jail right now. And as far as Oakland – best keep moving and let people sort out their own shit if you don't want a beat-down yourself."

"You're right," Stephan said in a resigned tone as he stared blankly out over the valley, "that kind of stuff is going on all the time. All we can do is try and turn around the fire experience and use it as motivation. Focus on our goals rather than wallowing in the misery of it all."

"You got it, brother. We both need to move on but when I see how I reacted to that guy torching himself I know I got a ways to go."

"Remember how the old-timers who planted the first orchards here called it 'The Valley of the Hearts Delight'? That's the spirit we need to reconnect with," Stephan said gesturing towards the vista spread out in front of them.

"And that's exactly why I call my outfit Eden. The whole India thing showed me that Edison did more to advance human evolution by inventing the light bulb than Karl Marx and Neem Karoli combined," James said. He stopped his pacing and stood facing Stephan and went on to explain that while he was sure he could make a positive influence on the world he was afraid of the price. The investor who funded their expansion from the garage at his parents' house to a floor of an office building had brought in a management team. James wasn't sure if they shared his vision and it concerned him. Stephan reminded him that the investor was buying into James's talent to translate a dream into products for a mass market that he had the near psychic ability to predict what would appeal to them. And the moneymen, even with a technical background, could only sense that possibilities existed. James grunted in acknowledgement and when Stephan went on to caution him against losing the connection to his human nature in trying to advance modern culture, James nodded wearily like it was his greatest struggle.

"See the rock over there with a notch in it?" James said nodding towards an irregular outcropping. "On the winter solstice the sun hits it and casts a shadow on that chunk of stone you're sitting on. The Ohlone believed your round rock represented a turtle that brought humanity back to earth after the big flood. It's all about cosmic cycles of birth, death and rebirth."

"Like Dylan said – those who aren't busy living are busy dying," Stephan said.

"You don't need a weatherman to know which way the wind blows. Dharma and karma."

"So what does the wheel of life tell you these days about Rosa? Still up and down, round and round?"

"I'm trying to figure it out. I think we're a perfect match, but after a year hanging out together she's dating another guy and doesn't want to see me anymore."

"What does your heart say?"

"I think she's an angel with devil's horns, a cold sun or something like a computer code: a one and a zero," James said.

"That last comparison was very romantic."

"Thanks. Every time I try to get closer she seems to move further away but I can't stop thinking about her."

James sat down again and plucked a length of wild grass he twirled around.

"You want my advice? You got to let go. Check out some other ladies because there are plenty of fish in the ocean. And a lot of them are just as cool and good-looking," Stephan said picking up a loose stone and tossing it down the hillside.

"Yeah, right," James said unconvinced.

Stephan told James that if he saw Rosa side-by-side with some other women, he'd see that there were more nice cute chicks around. And the day after tomorrow there was a big party in Saratoga at some kind of a new dance club called a disco and the guy who told him about it was a student at De Anza with Rosa and said she had agreed to go. Stephan was told he should bring some friends along and said to James it was a chance to check out Rosa alongside a bunch of other cuties.

James was thoughtful, digesting the words and then slowly lit up with a smile and agreed to the proposal. He stood and walked over to the solstice rock, putting his hand on the ancient marker, looking down at the bay. After a couple of minutes, he broke the contemplative silence they had drifted back into. "So when can I read some of this poetry you said you were working on?"

"It's not quite ready to share yet but I can give you a little taste." Stephan opened his cotton shoulder bag with a colorful ad in Sanskrit printed on the side, retrieved a notebook pulling out a folded-up piece of paper. "I call this 'Kabir's Blues'," he said flattening the page. He cleared his throat and spoke in an even tone.

"Death has got your number
But he ain't tellin' you
He's got ways to count your days
On one of them you're through
If you're feeling hungry
Now's the time to eat
'Cause there ain't no restaurant
Further down the street."

"Very cool, you nailed it," James said nodding in appreciation. "Kabir could talk about death in such a non-threatening way. And I like his ironic humor when he says the fish in the water is thirsty."

"That's right," Stephan said with a laugh. He switched to a more serious tone as he put away his poem. "I'm pulling all the notes together from those sessions with the silent baba so I can build them into my story."

"The wisdom of the East for the Wild West."

"Absolutely. Also, my old English Lit professor at Berkeley told me to show him the first couple of chapters because he can introduce me to a publisher if they are good enough."

"Excellent! Go for it, man. Let's see who can inspire a bigger audience – me with my thinking tools or you with your words."

"It's not a competition. I'm just trying to keep on the path and my book is helping me maintain the focus," Stephan said. "And last night I helped Greg teach a yoga class. We were talking and it looks like we're going to move over to Santa Cruz for a while."

"Sounds good. No rest for the karma bums." They both started laughing as the wind picked up and carried their laughter to the coast. "Look, you can see the Farallons," James said turning away from the valley view and pointing westward to where the Pacific spread like a copper-colored blanket dotted with patches of fog to the horizon. The distant islands appeared through the low clouds like ancient turtles rising from a primordial sea.

4

DISCO INFERNO

In 1976 the opening of the first disco in the South Bay was a major event that followed a shift from concerts with longhaired bands in converted ice-skating rinks to electronic music environments in stylized modern clubs with another kind of light show. No more squishy food colors beamed from an overhead projector onto a tie-dyed bed sheet – mirror balls and lasers were now the new environment of choice. The sweet smell of burning hemp was substituted by the scent of old socks as gay couples cracked open amyl nitrite for an instant high when not doing lines of coke in the bathroom. The novelty of pulsating lights, an illuminated dance floor and dozens of highly styled dancers created an alternative universe which was in part a celebration as well as a manifestation of a new, colorful hedonistic lifestyle. The disco craze had started as a black and gay underground scene and was reaching mainstream acceptance in the big cities as an alternative to rock music's increasingly loud punk and heavy metal direction. And now dance tracks were beginning to take Top Ten positions on the radio with artists like Gloria Gaynor, Hot Chocolate with 'You Sexy Thing' and the Silver Convention and their song 'Fly,

Robin, Fly', so it was only logical the phenomena would eventually reach the suburbs.

The boys were not too excited by the event itself but more curious to see what the new trend was all about and add it to their list of experiences. Greasy and Stephan had come over from Santa Cruz, rendezvousing with James at a party in the Los Gatos hills house of one of Greasy's acquaintances from his former life in Lake Tahoe. Bernie was the endless dealmaker with a short, round physique and was always trying to hustle something for a fast buck. Bernie knew Greg's friends and everyone else in the valley as his house had an open-door policy with a mix of guests in a continuous session of merrymaking where he supplied some of the materials for people to celebrate with for a modest fee. The party people made the drive over to the Odyssey Club on the Cupertino stretch of the Sunnyvale Saratoga Road in their usual mood of rolling chaos. Greasy was driving with one hand, guiding his prized metallic sea-green Chevy Impala with slant-six motor and push-button shifter, using his free hand to punctuate dialogue like an Italian caffeine addict. Stephan and James shared the backseat, and in the co-pilot position was a slim blond girl with long hair and a micro mini from the party Greasy had talked into coming along. Bernie followed them with some of his friends.

"So, James, this is your big chance. We're going to set you up with the stone fox to end all foxes. You're going to forget about Rosa once and for all," Greasy said with bravado and complete assurance.

"I wish it were that easy. I'm still really hung up on this lady."

"Time to move on. You've been moaning about her since she blew you off for that filmmaker dude. You're a hopeless romantic, my friend," Stephan said.

"We're going to help you out here, believe me. Beautiful women all shaking their cute butts, looking for the right hombre to take home," Greg said.

"Thanks, guys, I can look after myself."

"By putting a bikini a computer?" Greg said. Everyone laughed. His date slapped him playfully on the arm. "Hey, baby, don't worry – I'm not going to replace you with a box of blinking lights." Greg put his arm over the girl's shoulder squeezing her close. "Shiva/Shakti, AC/DC, yin and yang. We're all looking for a partner to feel complete but the other half is already inside," Greg said.

"Like a dog chasing its own tail," James said.

"Right on! We go crazy running in circles and never catch it in the end 'cause we already got it. But you have to admit there's nothing better than the celebration of cosmic union by getting tight with someone," Greg said.

"We are one in the spirit..." Stephan started to sing the old spiritual, laughing.

"A little tantra with my mantra if you know what I mean," Greg added, giving his lady another squeeze.

The disco was a swarm of people, searchlights and a non-stop stream of cars. They parked in a neighboring parking lot and joined the line in front of the entrance watched over by a couple of security guards that looked like off-duty football players. Bernie had dug up complimentary tickets somewhere, so they could all get in without paying. Once inside, Greasy steered his new lady friend through the crowd to the bar, while Stephan and James stood on the edge of the dance floor, watching the spectacle.

A fluid manifestation of the music in the form of a slinky dancer in a sparkling miniskirt instantly transfixed Stephan. She was so expressive of the nuances in the song that she became a physical extension of the pounding bass and swirling synthesizers. The dancer and the music were one, and Stephan blended into the oneness, watching her every motion, the flashes of light from the sequins on her tight dress accentuating the natural flow of her torso and long legs. A laser beam hit a large mirror ball on the ceiling, and the room exploded into a million sunrays tracing and illuminating the lithe body, and the dancer became the spirit of the disco, its soul and shimmering angel. She was uninhibited and one of the few people who were free of the rock-style dancing that most of the dancers clumsily adapted to the effervescent electronic beats.

Stephan turned to James who was scanning the crowd with his hands stuck deep inside the pockets of his jeans. "Please remind me that this vision is an innocent angel sent to inspire because there's a side of my brain telling me she's totally hot."

"You're a good yogi, I'm sure you'll find a way to deal with it," James said.

Stephan started to get lost again in his vision of an ethereal goddess and noticed James's attention being immediately drawn to a young lady on the edge of the crowd who looked like she was also in her early twenties. Her dark wavy hair was bound in a ponytail that accentuated her high cheeks and Latin looks while a black silk tank top and matching bell-bottomed pants flattered her youthful curves. Swinging her hips along to the beat, she eased onto the dance floor and joined in the party.

Stephan's show ended when a man in a flowery shirt with big lapels and white jeans whisked his disco doll from the dance area away to the bar. He turned his attention back to James and saw him follow the tall, dark lady onto the dance floor, separated by several groups of dancers and as people eventually edged off, he boogied closer trying to imitate the other dancers' moves. James looked entranced watching her as she moved fluidly to the music with an easy confidence. The lady acknowledged James with some direct glances as she checked out his dance moves. It was too crowded to get closer so it was up to the cosmic forces to align them. Stephan could see that James's course of antibiotics toned down his usual manic energy and assertiveness, so the usual direct approach was apparently not in his arsenal of seducers' tools this evening.

James focused on moving to the rhythm and every time he looked her way, she was watching him with an impish smile. The music switched to a song with a funky beat, and the DJ was shouting for the public to dance 'The Hustle'. James edged to the side of the crowd, embarrassed by his ignorance of the moves as couples joined in synchronized dance steps, the men with their polyester patterned shirts open to the navel and fat gold chains glinting against their chests. The public was elaborately styled with their colored bell-bottoms looking cool and trendy compared to James's dark jeans and black T-shirt. Some of the men wore bolero jackets with high lapels and one had what looked like an Italian spacesuit with metallic fabric and long tails that made James feel like the one who was an alien.

The music shifted back to some bass-dominated beats, and only a pair of gay men dancing together in platform shoes and white jumpsuits glowing under a black light separated James and the lady, who were now facing each other between the men. They shook, gyrated, and bounced to the beat, intent on each other as dance partners but not making eye contact. The music slowed, and the girl moved off the floor with James following discretely a few moments later.

Without warning she quickly disappeared into the crowd, so James roamed the bar area and Stephan joined him. They spotted Rosa, James's last love at the end of the bar with a cluster of other girls. James paused for a second not sure if he should approach her or not.

"You want to say hi?" Stephan asked.

James studied the group for a second before answering. "I'll survive. I think I've turned the corner."

"What did I tell you about checking some other ladies out? Looks like you found a new distraction on the dance floor."

"We'll see. And where's your dancing goddess?"

They circulated through the tables and James kept moving while Stephan joined Greasy where he was sitting at the bar, chatting with a bodybuilder in a white crew-neck shirt, black jeans and slicked-back hair who looked like Fonzie from *Happy Days*.

Greg was finishing a rap about the advantages of a slant-6 versus a V-8 cylinder layout, which met resistance from the buffed-out beer guzzler, who insisted his '57 Chevy was a triumph of engineering, especially with the modifications he had made.

"What's your name, man? I'm Greg Wheeler but everyone calls me Greasy."

"The name's Tobias DiFilippo."

"No kidding, is that your family who owns the trucking company?" Greg asked taking a drink from his beer.

"Yeah, that's us. Hauling tons of prunes a week for the Cappalettis and other farmers to ease the nation's constipated masses." They both laughed. "My old man also has some fishing boats over in Santa Cruz. But he's getting into investments and put up the money for this place."

"Cool. That makes you the manager or something?"

"Kind of." Tobias turned to the bar and waved at an older man in black turtleneck and jeans, hanging back in a small doorway between the rows of bottles on mirrored shelves. "Hey, Pops, I want you to meet someone."

The man broke away from the doorway he was supporting and seemed to slide over to the bar. He had dark eyes framed by bushy eyebrows and sagging ripples underneath while his wavy hair was receding and slicked back into a shiny shell.

"This is my new buddy, Greasy Greg, who claims to be one of the finest mechanics this side of Santa Cruz."

DiFilippo senior held out his hand for a quick handshake.

"Pleasure to meet you, Mr. DiFilippo. Fine establishment you've got here," Greg said.

"Thanks. How'd you hear out about this place?" he asked in a bored tone as he scanned the crowd.

"A friend of mine over there heard about it from some of his college friends." Greasy pointed to James standing at the edge of the dance floor. "He used to sell the students electronics gear, and now he has his own company building what he calls personal computers."

Tobias practically leapt off his barstool. "What? I don't want any of those technology bastards anywhere near this place. All they've done is ruin this valley for people like us. They have no respect for the land. I'm tossing his ass out."

"Hold on," DiFilippo senior cut in. "I don't want any problems on opening night. That young man has been behaving himself and is a cash-paying customer. His political or business interests don't matter tonight. What happens outside this place is another story, but let's not spoil the party."

"But Pop, you know as well as I do that it's either us or them."

"Just to let you know, my friend is actually a very ecology-oriented individual and wouldn't do anything to consciously hurt nature or the honorable profession of supplying the fruits of the earth," Greg said.

Tobias grabbed his beer and marched off to the back of the club, where he joined a group of equally burly colleagues.

Mr. DiFilippo shrugged his shoulders and said with the chill of an Antarctic iceberg, "The beer's on me. Enjoy your evening."

Stephan had been standing nearby with Greg's date watching the gyrating crowd, trying to spot his favorite disco doll while idly listening in with one ear to the car conversation between the two mechanics.

Stephan glanced at Greg and said, "Looks like James just lost a couple of sales." Greg laughed and his date returned to the bar, looping her arm in Greg's and pulling him to the dance floor while Stephan raised a beer in salute and watched the spectacle that once again included James's attempts to pursue his vision.

James had spotted the dancing lady with some friends in an open area between the bar and dance floor. He hovered nearby, casually leaning on a pillar looking in her direction for an opening. The lady kept turning and watching him and as he edged closer, she would look at him directly and part her lips as if to say 'here I am'. Stephan was amused as the normally fearless James looked like he was holding back due to a case of nerves. But then it began to make more sense: Rosa was at the bar watching him. Stephan could see the thought process like tiny cartoon bubbles over his head as James wondered if Rosa's attention signaled a possible rapprochement. James shook off the momentary confusion of conflicting thoughts and focused on the dancing lady with a sense of possibility. Stephan moved along looking for his glittering goddess.

James's new fascination turned away from her friends to face the dance floor, creating an opening so James moved close to her, also watching the dancers. When she looked in his direction and he turned, their eyes met and James, usually never at a loss for words, was paralyzed for an instant by a pair of hypnotic emerald green eyes.

She laughed at his predicament and spoke loudly over

the thumping music, "So you're a disco fan, are you?"

"You made a believer out of me," he shouted back to her amusement. James moved closer to not have to raise his voice too loud. "You're an amazing dancer."

"Not really, I just like to move to the rhythm."

"Are you from around here?" he asked with an inquisitive expression.

"Saratoga."

"I live in Cupertino, we're practically neighbors." The dancer laughed a shy nervous laugh in reply and turned to glance at her friends for a second.

"My name's James. What's yours?"

"Maria." She gave him a look that made him feel like an old friend.

"Nice to meet you," James said with an easy smile while Maria's eyes twinkled in response. "It's really loud in here, would you like to go outside?"

She nodded and he led the way to an inner courtyard that opened off the lounge area. A few couples were spread around the enclosed patio and he saw Stephan kicked back on a lounge chair idly watching the parade, half obscured by a bottlebrush plant with electric red blooms. They found an empty bench nearby and sat down.

"Can I ask you if you have Latin roots? You have a very exotic look," James said.

"Thanks. My family is Italian, if that's what you mean," Maria said while tossing her head proudly so that her hair cascaded over her shoulder.

"So that's why you're so stylishly dressed – do you model or do something in the fashion world?" James said trying to sound nonchalant.

"Nice try," she said smiling wisely at his line. "I express my personal visions through painting. And I get a lot of my inspiration from studying the images on tarot cards my Italian aunt taught me about."

"Wow, a gypsy fortune teller right here in Saratoga. Think I could get my future told sometime?"

"I think that could be arranged." Maria looked demurely at James, and before he could say anything, she gently took his hand with a naturalness that wasn't forced. He looked at her hand for an instant, surprised at its softness, and admired her exquisitely tapered fingers. "And what do you do?"

He told her about his company and its aims to revolutionize the way people work, play and communicate. He explained his ideals of empowering the everyman to help change the world with tools to do positive actions like writing and printing newsletters for community engagement. His company would reflect the philosophy of a new way to work as an example of an enlightened workplace run like a big family. Maria smiled bravely but looked disappointed. He asked what was wrong.

She gave his hand a squeeze of reassurance. "Just so you know, my father is Luigi Cappaletti. He's a local farmer who hates anything or anyone associated with these semiconductor companies."

"Uh-oh, I know that name. I'm on the anti-growth coalition's hit list. Are you supporting his cause?" James asked fearing the answer.

"Not entirely."

"Then I have some reason to hope."

"My dad and I don't always see eye to eye on things. He thinks my studying art is just an indulgence. And he also can't accept change which makes people like you his enemy," Maria said.

"I don't think anybody is programmed to accept change too easily."

"You're right." She deftly changed the subject while shifting her position on the bench. "And when I'm not painting I'm working towards a degree in art history at Stanford." She turned her body slightly to face him more directly. "But, you know, all the computer freaks I met there only talk about electrons and machinery. You're different."

"Maybe 'cause I'm also a sort of artist," he replied with a devilish grin.

Maria tilted her head slightly backward and to one side with half-closed eyes. The next thing James knew, he was leaning over and they were kissing. First, a soft gentle brushing of the lips leading to a gentle nibbling evolving to exploring tongues. They paused for a moment to come up for air and looked at each other like they were they only two people in the universe.

Someone calling from the door interrupted the reverie. One of Maria's girlfriends in a white blouse and short skirt was shouting across the patio. "Hey, Maria. We're leaving." Maria waved and then looked at James with big eyes, sadly indicating she had to go.

"Sorry, my dear James, fellow creative spirit, that's my cousin calling and it looks like the train is pulling out."

"Can I call you sometime? I would really like to talk with

you some more," James said taking both her hands in his.

"That would be nice."

"Are you in the phone book?"

"I am. You know my name and where I live, so I'm sure you'll figure out the rest."

She kissed him once more firmly and passionately and then slowly pushed herself away. She stood and walked across the patio while James got up and moved in the same direction in slow motion like a sleepwalking zombie who had missed a few days' slumber. Maria turned and waved over her shoulder while joining up with a group of friends heading towards the door. James noticed the muscle guy Greasy had been talking with was also in her crowd.

James found Greg finishing his beer at the bar and Stephan joined them. James had danced enough and without Maria there anymore, he was ready to leave.

"You sure picked the belle of the ball there," Greasy said.

"I know, she's beautiful, isn't she?"

"Get her phone number?" Stephan said. "You two looked quite friendly on the patio."

"Her dad is the Cappaletti that has me in his sights for the next farmer demonstration."

"Good move," Greasy said. He had his arm around his evening's date and smiled over his beer. "I was talking to the guy that hauls all her family's fruit around. He's a car freak from Santa Cruz. His family put up the bucks for this place, so you got to love him."

"If you hook up with her, you'll never have to worry about a shortage of fruit in your diet," Stephan said.

"Maybe her old man will hire you to pick apricots if

nobody buys any more of your electronics gear," Greasy said.

"Shut up. You're all just jealous," James said.

"Not me," Greasy said, swinging his date around with one hand over her head in a ballet pirouette, so she ended up with her back against his chest and his arm securing her across the waist. "Got my own little bundle of joy right here. And besides, I don't fancy your chances. When I told the trucker guy you were into circuit boards he got really uptight with some BS about the death of this valley. Looks like he's more of an environmentalist than you are, wonder boy."

"Thanks for the help. But don't worry, I'll still invite you to the wedding." They all laughed at his optimism and the image of James walking down the aisle.

Bernie rejoined them from one of his many rendezvous with various people he knew around the club and ordered a round for everybody. Greasy drank half his beer in one go and then steered his date onto the dance floor. James and Stephan took their drinks outside while Bernie chatted with a waitress.

"I can't believe this lady is real. She's so perfect – has a loving soul and really tuned in. She paints and is studying art. And she's really sharp – one of those Stanfordettes. I got so lost looking in those green eyes," James said as if he were stumbling along like an explorer in a deep jungle.

"Slow down, my friend, you just met her." Stephan twisted sideways to make space for a couple walking by in the small open area where they were standing on the patio.

"I know but there's something special there. I can feel it."

"I'd wait to order the wedding cake. Didn't you see how she left before midnight to show her parents what a good girl she is? She could have stayed and smooched some more if that was more important," Stephan said.

"That's your interpretation. You weren't sitting next to her."

"Did you see Rosa checking you out?"

"I did. And it was like… I can't explain it. She just didn't seem so important anymore, or the only woman in the world," James said and took a thoughtful sip from his juice.

"Thank God you got your head straight about that," Stephan said. "Anyway, let's see how you feel tomorrow. I'm curious if Rosa calls if you'll go out with her."

They went back inside and there was shouting and excited yelling from the dance floor. James looked at Stephan, and they spoke at the same time. "Greasy!"

They squeezed through the crowd in time to see Greg and his date in a simulated act of copulation, like two animated tantric love statues from an Indian temple. Greg released his partner's hips he had been grinding against and was on his knees, swinging his head back and forth in front of the girl's belly, keeping beat with the music with his tongue rapid fire flicking in and out like a snake, while caressing the backs of her thighs.

Suddenly two of the bouncers pushed their way through the circle of cheering spectators and grabbed Greg by either arm, lifting him up and pulling him off the dance floor. They walked Greg towards the door while he worked his jive talk into a friendly dialogue that ended with the bouncers laughing and slapping him on the back as they shrugged their shoulders as if to say it wasn't their choice he had to leave. The girl Greg was with saw James and Stephan and joined them, complaining that, even though they had been warned once, it wasn't fair because it denied them their freedom of expression.

They rounded up Bernie and left the club. James was stumbling, drunk on love with visions of the perfect woman.

"Sorry, Rosa, easy come, easy go," Greasy joked.

"Yeah, who will it be next week?" Stephan said.

Even Bernie, the Los Gatos Lothario couldn't resist a jab. "Look at you, useless!" Before their roasting could continue, the disco door burst open, banging against the front wall, narrowly missing the black-clad doorman. Tobias stood there for half a second and strode out, directly up to James.

"Hey, asshole," he said pushing James on the shoulder with his finger. "Maria's off limits."

"Cool it, man," Greasy said moving closer. "We're just having a good time, not bothering anybody."

"This doesn't involve you. This guy is making the moves on someone I consider family. He needs to know that it ends right here."

"It's only just beginning," James said coolly staring down Tobias taking some steam out of his aggressive tone.

"In your dreams," Tobias said, making a fist.

"Hey, take it easy, man," Greasy said, stepping beside Tobias. By now a couple of the trucker's friends had joined them and formed a semicircle behind Tobias as backup.

"I haven't done anything except talk with the lady. What's your problem?" James said.

"She's like my little sister and I'm watching out for her. In case you hadn't noticed, this whole goddamn valley is getting paved over with industry parks brought in by the likes of you." He pointed his index finger in James's face. "Her family made this valley into a paradise, and now you and your type are tearing the shit out of it putting people like me out of jobs." His words were accompanied by a mist of spray that James ignored. "You're wasting your time here. When Maria's old man finds out you're interested in her, he'll put an end to it."

"Sounds like this is more about incest than honor, mister big brother," James said. Tobias looked like he was going to explode, trying to find the right words to spit out while debating which form of physical violence to inflict. "I think you need to let Maria live her own life and not make her decisions for her," James added quickly.

"Go to hell. You don't get it." Tobias took a clumsy, drunken swing at James, but Greasy stepped in catching the arm. Tobias brought his left arm up but Greasy stepped back, still holding the right arm, pulling Tobias off balance.

"Hey, cool it," he said, releasing Tobias's hand. Tobias stood and glared at the group while his colleagues edged closer ready to spring.

"Like I said, it only involves me and you," Tobias said to James.

"Look, friend, we came and had a good time, but now we go in peace. No bad feelings," Greasy said.

Tobias looked directly at James. "I won't forget your face. Accidents happen." His friends laughed.

"Whoa," Greasy said. "Let's bring this back to planet

earth. Nobody's going to get hurt over a few words in a club."

Stephan interrupted the conversation. "Can't you guys settle this in a non-violent way like a race or something?"

"Yeah, right," Tobias said like it was the first sensible thing he had heard all night.

There was an awkward moment and then Greg chimed in. "You told me you had a hot car, right?"

"Smoking."

"Okay, so why don't we have us a little contest? I'll represent my buddy here, and if you win, he leaves your lady friend in peace, and if I win, you leave them alone to see what happens."

Tobias looked at him in bewilderment and then surprised everybody by saying, "You're on, greaseball."

Stephan saw James wasn't too happy to have someone else defend him but Greg had a way of defusing contentious situations and had done the compassionate thing knowing James was on antibiotics and only had an old VW bus.

They all agreed to meet several hours later at 3 a.m. when the roads were empty, racing from Saratoga village to Skyline Boulevard. Greasy had enough time to pick up his racer from Bernie's garage, where he had stored an odd collection of vehicles taken in trade for repair work. The '62 Porsche he rebuilt was his favorite. It needed some more work but basically it rolled. Tobias's Chevy was parked nearby in the VIP area and looked menacing in the harsh lights of the parking lot.

5

WHEEL OF FORTUNE

The stretch of Highway 9 that made up the racecourse was a short but challenging five miles of two-lane blacktop road twisting through redwood-lined ridges to the crest of the coastal mountain range. A group of cars filled a gravel turnout just outside the Saratoga city limits where the road disappeared into the forested hills and started its climb to eventually reach the coast.

Tobias's car was the most prominent. A two door '57 Chevy Belair hardtop with fins on the back from the tail of a Buck Rogers spaceship and a small pair of matching rocket nose cones recessed in the front hood. The rumble of the big block V8 engine, wide racing tires and metallic black paint job told everyone that this was a real muscle machine.

Greasy's 356 Porsche was like a toy in comparison, sitting next to the Chevy looking like a mutant VW Beetle with its light blue metallic paint. The extra suspension made it sit low to the ground and custom tubular steel bumpers gave the inverted bathtub shape a streamlined look. It also had a powerful motor modified for higher performance, located in the rear. With the traction and weight in the back the car tended to spin off the road backwards if the driver lost courage mid-turn and let up off the gas, allowing the powerful g-forces to pull the car engine first.

Greg's friend from mechanics school, a lanky teenager named Frank wearing a white T-shirt, worn-out Levis and waist-length ponytail was squatting barefoot by the engine compartment tuning the carburetor. Frank had helped rebuild the car so he knew the motor as well as Greg – and maybe even better as he practiced his trade day and night at his family's compound in the hills above Cupertino.

A representative was selected from each side to wait in the parking area at the summit to officiate the finish. Bernie represented Greg and had taken off ten minutes earlier, following a friend of Tobias named Boz. A couple more of Tobias's crew stood around, sizing up James and Stephan who were watching from beside James's VW bus. It was so beat-up looking it was a wonder it would roll, which was another reason James would have had no chance in a race. The two cars idled, with only the tall stands of bamboo in the Hakone Japanese gardens across the street as witnesses. It was damp and cool from the stream running alongside the road and the air had an organic stench from decomposing ferns and vegetation that rarely saw the light of day through the thick stands of laurel trees.

"You think you can beat me in that VW?" Tobias called over to Greg.

"You're going to be surprised when all you see is my dust."

Tobias tossed his empty beer can off into the bushes, where it clanked against its empty brother and stepped closer to the Porsche. "I'll try and notice if I accidentally drive over you 'cause you won't be bigger than a bump in the road to me. Hope you got a roll bar in that little tin can for when you go bouncing off some redwood trees."

"You won't get close enough, so save your breath," Greg answered, easily dismissing the threat.

"If you're so fucking confident, let's race for the pink slips – winner takes all. Your propeller head friend doesn't stand a chance anyway with Maria, so let's at least make it interesting."

"You're on," Greg said, grinning. They slapped hands in a modified handshake.

"When I win that wreck of yours, I'll gonna junk it at the bone yard just for the hell of it. Wouldn't be caught dead driving a tub like that – looks like something my little sister would drive." He and his crew laughed. "Okay, let's do it," Tobias said. He walked back to his car stretching his arms, climbed in and revved the engine.

Greg approached James and Stephan who were still standing by James's bus. James said, "Take it easy, man. This isn't worth getting hurt over."

"I'm just an instrument of higher forces. It's the same to me whether I win or lose but I sure ain't going to let my baby go without a fight." He punched James on the shoulder, slipped Stephan a soul shake and then held his open hand low, facing up.

"Give me five. Five will get you ten," Greg said like a ghetto pimp.

Stephan slapped the hand in response. "Flow with the go, brother."

Frank closed the engine compartment letting the cover

fall with a solid clunk and gave Greg a thumbs-up signal. Greg walked back to his car and climbed in, gunning the engine. The deep-throated roar showed it had once been a standard motor, but some serious modifications had made it a beast.

The two cars lined up side by side on the road, alternately revving their engines and rocking forwards and backwards as each driver found the balance point for the clutch. It was just after three in the morning, so no other traffic was on the highway. They would have heard any vehicles coming down from the summit, and no cars had passed in the last fifteen minutes heading to the top. The motors hummed with an occasional grinding growl when the driver gave a little gas to increase the idle range. The Chevy rumbled and looked like it would pull half the road along with it on take-off. The Porsche had a rhythmic, pounding sound exaggerated by the sport exhaust – just an enlarged pipe with no muffler to stifle the performance.

One of Tobias's friends stood on the gravel shoulder and raised his hands as the two cars revved their engines. On one hand he held up five fingers and lowered them one by one, and with the last finger folding, dropped both hands. There was a terrific screaming of rubber on tarmac with blue smoke pouring from the spinning back wheels of each car.

Greasy was faster on the start, springing forward in a flash, but the Chevy blasted off, chasing the tail of the Porsche. Tobias pulled even on the short straightaway with his wheels still smoking and in the first curve all but pushed the Porsche off the road. Greasy braked as the Chevy surged ahead and he kept the pressure up, tailing the Chevy and forcing Tobias's car into even more risky turns.

The road switch-backed as it made the ascent, twisting left and right like a slinky snake. In every hairpin turn Greasy would edge around to pass, as his car was more maneuverable. But Tobias always nosed over, and if Greasy hadn't braked, he would have been crunched against the hillside or run off the road into one of the steep ravines full of scattered granite outcroppings.

The two cars raced higher, Tobias powering his machine upward with the extra horsepower chewing up the miles with no effort. Greasy followed closely and finally, on a banked curve, Greg shot past with his motor whining at the high RPM it took to get the necessary passing speed. Tobias cursed and tailgated Greg mercilessly. All Greasy saw in his rearview were the grinning chrome grill and big headlights looking like some Oriental demon ready to consume him in one ferocious bite. Sliding too wide into a curve, Greg cursed as he gave enough of an opening for the Chevy to blast by.

Greg kept up the pressure by faking passes left and right anywhere he could. They had covered half the distance, and the view of the valley that flashed by on the east-facing turns was the dazzling wattage of endless streetlights like an upside-down futuristic sky.

Frustrated by the Porsche constantly pestering him, Tobias gunned the car on a straightaway, not caring that a hairpin turn was 100 yards ahead. Greg accelerated quickly, and his lights soon filled Tobias's back window. The signs with U-shaped black arrows on a white background indicating a sharp turn flashed by, ignored by both drivers. The posted speed limit was thirty, but both cars were doing over twice that.

Greg quickly downshifted; approaching the turn to use the top end of second gear with the higher RPM to slingshot him past the Chevy. Tobias kept up his speed, and as Greg faked a move to the left to get a gap on the right to pass, Tobias again swung left to block the way. Tobias moved too far over, entering the curve. His left rear wheel slid onto the gravel and dirt shoulder, momentarily losing traction. The Chevy's tail started to slide sideways as he spun out, with one wheel gripping the road and the other flying at a different speed, with nothing solid to hold onto in the soft shoulder.

Tobias turned the wheel hard to the right to counter the out-of-control movement, but at the speed he was going, compensated too much. The car lurched and with enough sideways motion began to roll. It flipped quickly on its back, sliding rear end first to the other side of the road. The weight and momentum carried the car over the small embankment and with no guardrail it disappeared swiftly over the edge of a steep hillside, rolling a couple of times crashing through brush and flattening small scrub oak and manzanita bushes in its path. With the last rotation the Chevy came to a rest on its roof at a forty-five-degree angle against a large boulder with a final loud crash.

Greasy hastily hit the brakes to avoid hitting the car as it swept sideways in front of him, downshifted and braked some more to reach a complete stop. He backed up at full speed to the turnout where the Chevy had disappeared, and parked. As Greg got out, he could hear a couple of cars racing down from Skyline Boulevard a half mile away. The people at the top had heard the cars approaching, the crashing noises followed by the sound of only one car and then silence.

Greg was halfway down the hillside, scrambling through the thick brush, careful to avoid a tumble to the bottom of the steep ravine. As he made his way to where the car rested, Bernie shouted down to him from the road. Greg didn't reply but kept on as fast as he could, focused on reaching the car. The Chevy's roof was flattened almost level with the hood and the doors were wedged shut with all the glass broken out. Some of the safety glass from the front window hung in clumps over the hood.

There was an eerie silence only disturbed by Bernie and the trucker's friend crashing through the chaparral, while Greg surveyed the scene. He carefully skirted the car to see if there was a way in or if Tobias had managed to jump out and was lying nearby. Looking uphill at the path the car had carved through the terrain a flash of white caught his eye off to the side about twenty feet away. He pushed his way through the thick tangle of brush and found Tobias lying on his side with his head bent at an exaggerated angle from a broken neck. Moving to the front of the body he could see Tobias's face was heavily scratched with his eyes open, staring straight ahead. The pressure from the impact had caused internal bleeding and a few of drops of blood escaped from the lower corner of each eye forming two trails of red tears across his cheeks.

When the two race marshals joined Greg and saw the body, the three of them stood around in shocked silence not sure what to do. Greg took off his jeans jacket and gently covered the head and upper body.

"Can one of you go and call for some help?" Greg said with his voice about to break, still watching the body.

Boz sat heavily on a small boulder repeating, "Oh my God," in hoarse whispers, not believing what had happened. He said Tobias's name slowly a couple of times as if it would bring him back to life.

"You okay, man?" Bernie asked Greg putting a hand on his shoulder.

"Just go and get some help," was the only reply delivered in a defeated tone as Greg turned and stared at the crumpled car below. Bernie immediately took off up the hillside and headed back up to Skyline, where the closest payphone was to call for an emergency crew.

Greasy was sitting on a rock sobbing when James and Stephan found him. He looked like he was in a state of shock, rocking back and forth, talking to himself.

"Hey, buddy, you alright?" Stephan said kneeling next to him.

"I can't believe this is happening. A couple of hours ago we were talking car bullshit, and now he's dead. It was so stupid to race the guy."

"You're not to blame," James said. "It could have been you."

"Thanks, friend, real consoling words. If it wasn't for your dick he'd still be alive." Greg was looking at the ground with an expression of frustration and anger.

"Hold on," Stephan said, "nobody is to blame here. This was an accident. Tobias knew his car and besides, he was drunk. We all saw that. He pushed the limit once too much."

"Doesn't bring him back now, does it?" Greg said quietly looking up and staring at Stephan.

Boz, who had been sitting nearby looking stunned, got up and stumbled over the rough, slanted landscape. Leaning to one side, to compensate for his top-heavy bodybuilder frame, he confronted Greg.

"You're going to get it, punk, I'll see to that." The young man paused, and he was sobbing again. He walked a few yards away and sat dejectedly on the ground with his head between his knees. Two other of Tobias's friends who had just arrived stood nearby surveying the accident and lifeless body, unsure what to do.

A series of intertwining wails pierced the silence, gradually growing louder as if reality was approaching to bring the inhabitants of the surreal scene back to planet earth. An ambulance, fire department vehicle, two Highway Patrol cars and a mountain rescue team arrived, flagged down by Bernie who had returned from the summit. They parked along the road with their red and blue flashing lights flickering over the landscape of twisted scrub like strobe lights. Frank was also waiting by the road after a quick look at the wreck and had been examining the skid marks trying to understand the cause of the accident.

Two ambulance attendants carefully carried the body up the hill on a stretcher after the Highway Patrolmen had examined the scene. The patrolmen were taking statements, and as the only actual witness, Greg was grilled where he sat in the backseat of a cruiser with a blanket over his shoulders to dull any effects of shock. After Greg finished giving his account, the police decided to temporarily impound the Porsche, so Greg rode with Bernie back to the valley while Stephan followed with James in his bus. Frank had said his goodbyes and left ahead of them flying down the hill in an ancient Dodge pickup.

Stephan was staring straight ahead into the tunnel of trees lit by the van's headlights; only moving when the bus jerked forwards when James shifted gears. They were halfway down to the valley when James finally spoke.

"I can't believe that guy is dead."

"Maybe we're dreaming," Stephan said putting one hand on the dashboard so he didn't slide along the seat. "I feel like this isn't really happening. Life and death are so close."

"Somehow it's like what we saw in India – something so unreal."

"At least in India we could see what was going to happen, so it wasn't a total shock," Stephan said.

"But tonight, I wish we would have stopped the race."

"We sure would have if we knew what the outcome was going to be," Stephan said scanning the lights in the valley below as they made another turn.

"It blows my mind to think that one minute there's a hoodlum waving his fist in your face, and a few hours later he's gone, forever. It's like watching a movie and when the lights come up, it's over."

"I thought I was suggesting a way to avoid some violence, and instead someone died," Stephan said.

"Don't blame yourself, everyone acted on their own." James paused to concentrate on piloting a tight curve. "It's also so weird to think that I met somebody special and had such an amazing connection, like she could really be the one, and then this happens."

"What I can't believe is that it was my idea to have the damn race," Stephan said.

"Forget about it." James looked at Stephan to make his point and there was a silence as they both watched the road roll by.

They had reached the Saratoga village and turned south on the Saratoga–Sunnyvale Road towards Los Gatos and were soon at Bernie's old Victorian house, where all the lights were blazing as if to scare off any ghosts lingering in the vicinity.

Inside the rustic wood-paneled living room, Greg was sprawled on the beat-up sofa, with his feet stretched out on a low coffee table and his arms crossed on his chest, staring into space while his date was curled up in an armchair opposite, watching him with a worried look. They could hear Bernie on the phone in the kitchen, checking in with his network to see what the buzz was on the street.

"Hey, what's going on?" Stephan asked as he and James sat on a second beat-up plaid sofa that was at right angles to Greg.

"I don't know, everything and nothing," Greg said in a weary tone.

"Look, I'm so sorry about what happened, it shouldn't

have been you in the middle," James said.

"Thanks, but the deal is done. The dude's wasted."

"It was obviously not your fault. Someone who drank too much is a risk to themselves and anyone else that's around," Stephan said.

"You guys want to hear what happened?" Greg said in a stronger tone looking at his two friends. They nodded, attentive to his story. He described how the two drivers were racing like crazy with Tobias trying to run him off the road whenever Greg would make a move to pass. Greg was on his tail when they came to the big bend towards the top and Tobias lost control on the soft shoulder. He tried to counter-steer but that trick only works on a dirt track when all the wheels are on the same surface, so he slid into a four-wheel drift and flipped the car.

"Yeah, but listen to what you're saying," Stephan said. "He was trying to run you off the road. Which means he was looking to kill you. And he died trying!"

"He might have made it if he hadn't downed so many beers and pushed the limits," James added.

"We'll never know, will we?" Greg said as he sat up straight folding his legs under him. "Hey, guys, I appreciate your checking in on me, but there's not much else we can do tonight. Let's hook up tomorrow and see what the world looks like. And my new friend here is still in a state of shock. Come here, baby," Greg said, extending an arm towards the young lady.

After a short, fitful sleep, James had been debating if he should call Maria or not and finally around two in the afternoon decided to try and reach her. Waiting through half an hour of busy tones, James finally got her on the phone. Figuring she'd already heard the news he gave his condolences but Maria sounded exhausted and distant. She explained that her whole family was in a state of shock and both her father and Tobias's had been at the police station wanting Greg arrested and sent to the electric chair. They claimed the blood test was tainted that said Tobias had twice the legal level of alcohol as well as the breathalyzer test that cleared Greg. The DiFilippo family was not only longtime partners but somehow distantly related, like many Italian families are, so the event was treated like a family matter. Mr. DiFilippo was swearing revenge in the old Italian way of an eye for an eye. Maria told James that if his friend valued his safety he better leave town.

The call was cut short when someone picked up an extension. There was only one phone line in Maria's house, so James had no chance to propose a meeting before Maria said a quick "bye" and hung up. He sat in a preoccupied funk in his office nursing a feeling of loss and emptiness. Reflecting on the call he saw it was insensitive of him to have called someone he barely knew at a time of a personal tragedy. But he also couldn't stop himself because he had been continually thinking about her since they met. James telephoned Bernie's house and told Greg about the danger he was in and encouraged him to lie low, ideally in another city.

Stephan showed up a while later after James had called, and discussing Maria's warning with Greg and Bernie, they looked at the options. It was clear Greg needed to leave town for a while until things cooled off. Tahoe was out, too near, same for Marin County. Santa Cruz wasn't an option as it was the DiFilippo family home base so that ruled out anywhere along the coast between Big Sur and San Francisco.

Greasy momentarily revived from his quiet state to show he had been listening to Stephan's points. "Listen up. I've got a long-standing offer from an old friend turned film producer in LA to be his personal mechanic. The guy has a Mercedes, a Mini Cooper plus a couple of Porsches. It's probably the only option going."

Stephan considered what the future might hold for his good friend and then heard himself say, "Maybe I'll join you. I always wanted to check out the scene in Southern California. We can teach our yoga classes in LA just as easily as in Santa Cruz. And who knows, maybe my Rama story could be your producer buddy's next film."

Greg laughed, breaking his somber mood. "And who will you get to play the lead role? Warren Beatty?"

"I was thinking Peter Fonda would be good. No, really, I'm ready for a change. I'm tired of sharing a big house with a bunch of crazy students who continually eat my food and wake me up at all hours with their loud music."

Bernie said he would buy the Porsche, so Greg would have some cash to keep him going, and if he ever wanted it back, the option was always open. The next morning before first light Greasy and Stephan returned to Santa Cruz, packed their few belongings, and headed south.

6

WELCOME TO LA

The drive to Los Angeles felt more like an exodus than a new beginning for Stephan and Greasy. The weather accentuated the feeling, being typically gray for this time of the year, as the late summer gave way to the cool mornings of an approaching fall, with a low fog that created a gloomy atmosphere for the forced change. The two exiles had each tossed a duffle bag and backpack with their few belongings in the trunk of a beat-up Impala, along with Greg's toolboxes, and started driving early on Monday morning. They headed south from Santa Cruz on the Coast Highway passing endless fields of artichokes, turning inland just before Monterey to eventually pick up 101, where it passed through Gilroy. They drove by the Laguna Seca Raceway where Greg had planned to race his Porsche in an antique car race that coincided every year with the Pebble Beach Concourse of Autos. But it served as only a stark reminder of the accident instead of an ambitious goal.

Stephan didn't remind Greg that James Dean, the teen idol from the fifties film *Rebel Without a Cause*, was on his way to the same track when he wrecked his Porsche nearby, killing himself. No sense reviving the image of a fallen hero who lived too fast and died too young – as Greg seemed to be doing, Stephan thought. Inspired by the raceway, Greg started a fast-talking monologue on the racing exploits of Mario Andretti, recounting his Indy 500 races and getting excited when he gave a lap-by-lap replay of the famous 1975 Spanish Grand Prix where Andretti had qualified fourth and led for nine laps before his suspension failed. Stephan was happy to see a spark of the old Greg appear, as this type rap had been one of his earlier trademarks from his days with Neal Cassady. Stephan was in awe of the times Greg had spent with Cassady as *On The Road* was one of his favorite books that he had read and reread a dozen times. Once more, as he had many times in the past, he got Greg going on the subject of finding the cool place inside and another fifty miles flew by.

As the acres of freshly tilled farmland rolled past, Stephan was trying to put the whole chain of events together in his head to understand how they had come to this juncture and hoped it was part of his personal evolution. They were mostly silent, as the racing incident was still too fresh. Yet with an eight-hour drive the subject would occasionally pop up, as there wasn't much scenery to distract them and the radio kept fading in and out as they passed out of range of one broadcaster after another. They had taken another jog eastward to Interstate 5, which was one long, straight road through the Central Valley, which would make their drive south faster. The landscape was flat and empty with not much more than ploughed fields and the low, squat buildings of vast chicken farms to look at, as a foggy haze had dimmed any prospect of viewing the monotonous rolling foothills on either side of the broad expanse of open land.

"So how long has it been since you last saw your producer buddy?" Stephan asked.

"When you were in India we had a Tahoe reunion and rented a big old Victorian for a week. Made some peyote tea and some musicians from San Fran jammed all night. That's when Bill told me he could use my help."

"You sure he wasn't tripping too heavy when he said that?"

"Talked to him yesterday to be sure, and got directions so we're all set," Greg said as if this had been their plan for many months.

"Cool. Will be good to have someone to show us the ropes. I remember LA being this huge spread-out mass of concrete covered with freeways."

"You just got to know where it's happening. Lot of groovy people."

"You think being in LA will help us get beyond what happened?" Stephan said looking at Greg from where he slouched in the corner of the front seat.

"Don't know. Right now there's a lot of stuff mixed together. James is a soul brother who's brought change."

"He's sure the whole mess is his fault."

"It sort of is, but then he wasn't driving the car," Greg said.

"Take it easy. You know as well as me the Chevy was a street racer not a rally car like your Porsche."

"But if I hadn't agreed to a contest, the guy would still be around," Greg said.

"And if there had been no race – a fight in the parking lot with broken heads and ugly faces? And another next week."

There was a pause in the conversation as Greg concentrated on overtaking a couple of tractor-trailer rigs. "It's hard to accept someone died and I was the cause. When you read about an accident in the paper it's impersonal and just another sad loss. But when it's someone you were connecting with on a certain level and then later pushing them 'til they went beyond their limits, I can't help but feel some blame."

"It could have just as easily been you getting measured for a coffin," Stephan said.

"But it wasn't."

"There was no intent for anyone to get hurt so you weren't acting in a bad way. Besides, a race is the wrong way to settle an argument. If I had kept my mouth shut we would all be better off."

"Now don't you get started. We both have to make our peace with what happened. Like Credence said – the 'big wheel keeps on turning', so let's keep rolling down the river and see what's next. Maybe you'll even find a replacement for your cute yoga lady from the bakery. You all seemed real tight for a while, but wait 'til you see the fine ladies on Sunset Strip!"

Greg wasn't too bothered by such details as commitment and had slept his way around Santa Cruz with a variety of willing ladies, ranging from stylish hairdressers to bored housewives to mystical mamas in love beads and India print skirts stinking of patchouli oil. Love was to be shared with no hang-ups or concepts please.

Stephan failed to answer as he drifted off in a trip down memory lane thinking back to the blond student from the bakery and her silky smoothness and sweet smells. Greg turned up the radio and started singing along to 'Sweet Home Alabama' and used his arms in the exaggerated gestures of an Indian dancer doing a Shiva temple dance.

A few miles later, when the radio signal faded out, Greg asked Stephan if he was able to get back to work on his book.

"The best I could manage is a first chapter. I sent it off last week to that underground paper, *The Oracle*, up in the city."

"Cool, you have to let me read it. Remind me what it's all about."

"At the end of the day it's the same old story – two dudes fighting over a girl. The root of all evil and all that."

"Where have I heard that before?" They both laughed. "Don't you think the story of Krishna is better? That guy had a thousand milkmaids in love with him and made a copy of himself for each of them. That's hot – people want sex, and he was like Hugh Hefner – king of the bunnies."

Stephan shared the outline of the story explaining how Rama was a prince who was cheated out of becoming king by an evil stepmother and banished for a dozen years. Rama, his beautiful wife and his devoted brother lived in a wild forest and helped the local monks and sadhus by getting rid of some demons, one of which was the sister of an evil king. For revenge and also because of falling in love with Rama's wife, the evil king kidnapped the wife.

After many adventures and help from a monkey army the princess was rescued. Rama finally returned home and became the king. Stephan was adapting it to a more modern version with the son of a wealthy businessman moving to the ghetto with his wife and brother, cleaning out the gangs before encountering a Mafia boss who steals the son's wife. The tale of unjust banishment and triumphant homecoming gave the two friends hope that their exodus would also have a return chapter.

The weather improved as they moved further south, with the flat gray ceiling breaking up to reveal a brilliant blue sky. There were long, low clouds in animal shapes moving like a caravan behind the coastal range. They came back to the Coast Highway just above Santa Barbara where the rolling green foothills from the Santa Ynez Mountains extended to the flatlands above the beach like toes on a giant foot. They cruised down the palm-tree-lined highway close to the ocean where surfers and oil rigs were visible offshore and eventually made their way back inland towards Camarillo, home of the sanitarium where Charlie Parker cleaned up his heroin habit in the middle of his bebop career. Climbing the last ridges before the upper end of the San Fernando Valley, the clear coastal air became tinged with a golden-brown color as the smog overflowing from the LA area forced its way north. They were on the 405 Freeway now and passing through the early beginnings of a nascent suburban sprawl. From 'The Valley' they followed the 405 over the Cahuenga Pass and at the crest exited on Sunset Boulevard.

The fabled road twisted its way eastward towards Hollywood passing through the green-forested grounds above UCLA before entering the genteel outer reaches of Beverly Hills where massive lawns fronted Spanish and Mediterranean-style villas in commanding positions. Sunset was meandering in a civilized manner along an immaculately manicured meridian, when, on the left side, they passed the Beverly Hills Hotel in its entire pink art deco splendor. The boulevard started to enter West Hollywood with the first of the high-rises looming over them: the Playboy building with the famous bunny logo on the top. Swanky restaurants and huge billboards advertising rock bands and movies became the new landscape. By now the air was thick and smelling of sulfur, visible like a low fog a block ahead of them. The windows were rolled down because of the heat and their eyes burned. Greg found a local rock station on the radio for an appropriate soundtrack to accompany their tour. They passed the Rainbow and Roxy clubs before driving by the Whisky A Go Go, and as the street started to straighten and the rows of hookers began to appear they turned away from the Hollywood Hills and headed down towards the LA basin.

They located the production company's offices on Larchmont Boulevard, just south of Melrose, in a quiet area that was half residential, interspersed with small businesses. The small Spanish-styled houses were once in a permanent siesta on a sleepy side street with the biggest activity being the sprinklers going on at night to water the perfectly manicured front lawns. Due to the close proximity to the major studios some of the homes had become production offices.

A colorful sign that could have been advertising a real-estate office announced they were at Authentic Films. A short slogan in smaller letters 'The Reel Thing' accompanied the ornate name on the hanging slab of wood in front of a large white bungalow complex. Inside, the offices were modern, with a black and chrome décor and, mercifully, air-conditioned. There was no receptionist at the desk in the entry to greet the two travelers, but out of the flow of casually dressed people going in and out of the various rooms they managed to find someone who knew Greg's friend. They were invited to hang out in the lounge area until the producer showed up.

The buzz of activity from clacking typewriters and phone calls created a background noise that was supplemented by the repetitive whine of unintelligible rewound dialogue from an editing room along the main hall. The previously garbled words followed correctly when the film played back from the starting point one more time. The two guests looked in the room where a large editing machine with multiple rolls of 35mm film that endlessly stopped, rewound and started again, displaying images on a grainy monitor in front of the editor wearing a colorful silk scarf and electric blue T-shirt who busily marked and cut the film.

There was an endless stream of people passing through the lounge/living room where they waited observing that the dress code dictated mainly T-shirts and jeans for both sexes. Greasy was restless and wired from the eight-hour drive and paced the room like a caged tiger, getting endless cups of water from the cooler. Stephan was content to sit on the black leather sofa and read the industry news in a copy of *Variety*, hiding his awkwardness of being in a strange office without any agreed agenda.

Greg greeted everyone walking by with "howdy" and "hey man", getting a few laughs from the ladies, who liked his directness when he said "how ya doin', ma'am" with a mock tip of his hat like a country boy in the big city.

Half an hour later, an animated man in his thirties dressed in a white collarless dress shirt and tight faded jeans came in, and seeing Greg, broke into a grin and smothered him in a bear hug.

"Let's look at you, man!" The guy pulled away and held Greg by each shoulder looking him up and down. He had dark shoulder-length hair that was stylishly cut and wore some silver and turquoise jewelry with a hipster's flair. Greg introduced Stephan to the producer, whose name was Bill, and they shook hands.

"Been a while since Tahoe, eh man?" Bill said grinning at some mutual unspoken joke.

"Lifetimes. Looks like you've done okay for yourself," Greg said, nodding to the plush offices.

"Not too bad. Making films is really a trip. You'll see – I'll take you guys out to the set tomorrow and you can check it out. And you being the ladies' man, will really dig these babes. Hey, but no pimping, all right?"

"No problem, I'll just admire the scenery. Besides, I came down here to work on other chassis than just them nubile young women. I'm into wrenches not wenches."

"We'll see. When you get your rap going about kundalini

rising through the chakras and eternal union, they just line up for your private yoga classes with their panties soaked in anticipation. That's why I had to leave Tahoe – never had a chance."

"So where are all these hot rods that need fixing? You told me you're always getting ripped off and needed a trustworthy mechanic."

"It's great you're here, my babies are in need of some real TLC."

"I'm your man, slick. My buddy Stephan came along to check out the City of the Angels and if you need someone to carry shit around on a film set or something, he's the one. He did some of that in college for an artsy student film with wizards and dragons. He's also a hot-shot writer, so might even have a story for you one day."

"Groovy," Bill said. "We'll put you both to work right away. And I guess you need a place to crash?" He looked at them with raised eyebrows and Greg nodded affirmatively. "A couple of the crew have a big house not far from here and would rent you country bumpkins a room if you don't mind parties, groupies, drugs, sex and rock 'n' roll. There's a garage out back I rented for you to set up shop in. In between working on my babies, you could do tune-ups on some of my friends' cars and make a few extra bucks."

"Sounds cool," Greg said beaming like he just won the lottery. Stephan watched the two friends' exchange from where he was getting some water at the cooler, not sure what he was getting into.

"Hey, I was kidding about the party scene. These guys at the house are actually serious vegetarians, so you might even get some healthy food and not that diet of nachos and beer you usually start the day with."

"I'm not sure I'm going to like this. What did you think we came here for, to be saints?" Greasy said.

"It's never too late, man. Look, I got a meeting here in an hour, so why don't you go and check out the place, and then we'll meet back here tomorrow morning at ten and get you started. I'll drive down there with you and make the intros."

The house was on a small side street parallel to Wilshire Boulevard, a few blocks from Western Avenue, where a once respectable middle-class neighborhood was unsuccessfully fighting a slow slide into seediness. The landlords didn't care about maintaining the houses as long as the rent came in, so the front yards were generally weedy or scattered patches of grass from lack of water, and the paint was faded or else peeling. While most houses on the street were family dwellings, where a sense of permanence was nurtured, a couple of them were rented to students or communal arrangements.

Greg and Stephan's future residence was a three-story house fronted by a barren front yard with occasional clumps of dried-out crabgrass and a pillared front porch piled full of shoes. It wasn't much different than the other houses along the stretch of street with the exception of a few further down that the original owners actually lived in and maintained with a more kept-up look. The dirt driveway along the side of their house led to a two-car garage and small backyard with an abandoned kids' playground set. Greasy eyed the rusty swing-set frame as the future home for a winch to pull engine blocks out of cars.

The housemates were agreeable and operated as a semi-commune. It was a mix of four men and an equal number of women, who ate their meals together. A part of the shared rent paid for food and the support of a lady who cooked and took care of the household. It was a democratic arrangement with a bright-eyed guy in his late twenties named Barry with close-cut hair, who acted as a leader to focus issues that were either on-going or occasionally cropped up. He encouraged a vegetarian, non-smoking lifestyle based on his studies of yoga, raw-foods dieting and desert fasting – something Greg and Stephan were used to, so they were rapidly accepted.

The other roommates were in their early twenties and either working for studios or had day jobs to support their migration from the Midwest to the land of endless sunshine and impossible dreams. Stephan and Greg were shown a small room on the first floor, where they could roll out their sleeping bags. The Santa Cruz exiles were replacing two tourists from Lebanon and Switzerland that had spent a couple of months hanging out in LA until their visas had run out.

Within an hour of unpacking and gobbling down some leftovers, Greasy was already in the kitchen, rapping with the lady housekeeper. She was a cute blond from Minnesota in a granny dress, happy to be able to experience an alternative lifestyle more open than what her conservative home offered. Stephan looked in for a moment, listening to their discussion. Greg had been praising her cooking, telling her the cuisine was good enough for a restaurant.

The housekeeper thanked him and sighed. "My lower back's killing me. I think I've been standing around too long."

"I know exactly what the problem is," Greg said.

"You do?" she replied quietly with a hint of hope.

"It's clear. Your lower chakra is blocked. What you need is an orgasm."

Stephan had been leaning against the wall listening and was embarrassed at Greg's casual straightforwardness but then, after stacking a couple more rinsed plates in the dish rack, the housekeeper said, "You think that's all it is?"

Stephan walked up to a coffee shop on Wilshire with one of the guys that worked as a production assistant on Bill's film crew. Stephan wanted to get some idea of what was expected and was told that, while not too stimulating intellectually, the money was good. The job title was a glorified name for a slave of all trades that hauled backdrops and equipment from one set-up to the next.

When Stephan returned to his room an hour later, he instinctively opened the door quietly and through the small crack could see in the dim candlelight Greasy and the cook lying side by side under a blanket in an act of mutually applied oral sex. He quietly closed the door and went downstairs to the living room to read a magazine until he heard the lady climb the stairs twenty minutes later to the room she shared with another woman on the top floor.

Bill gave them an early morning tour of the set, where a movie he was producing for a television network was having some scenes shot. The film was a romantic comedy about a boss and his secretary's Cinderella-like transformation, with some middle-tier TV stars stumbling through their lines, acting out a scene in an office set-up. Bill got Stephan signed onto the production crew and then disappeared with Greg to get him started on the first of many repairs.

Stephan's first day on the job was exactly like what he had been told – helping a couple of crew members on a soundstage set up for scenes by moving ten-foot tall wooden frames that held painted canvas scenery depicting exotic landscapes. The low-budget production was being shot at Producers Studio, a broken-down film lot just off Melrose, opposite the south gates of Paramount. The crew was friendly, and while the work was hard, Stephan was excited to be on the set of an actual film even though it was only for television.

A couple of weeks later Stephan was in the studio commissary that had doubled as a Wild West canteen for some 1950s Westerns, having a discussion over lunch with one of his housemates named Ray, who was also working on the film. The initial excitement and glamour had worn off, and Stephan was trying to see a way forward.

"You know, this manual labor is a good, non-thinking activity that suits a yogic lifestyle," Stephan said.

"Yeah, and I don't mind steering clear of building up a big ego to survive in a corporate environment. And besides, the money is really decent," Ray said.

"For sure. It's the most I've ever been paid. And with all this heavy work I get a good sleep at night, but somehow it isn't enough." Stephan pushed his plate away that still had some remnants of a Mexican meal. "I guess I'm frustrated because my writing is on hold for the moment. I want to get back to work on my book but the days here are always so long and there's no real privacy at the house for working with the concentration I need."

"I hear you. I got a screenplay I'm developing. Remember that old TV show called the *Little Rascals*?"

"Sure, *Our Gang* with Spanky, Buckwheat and Alfalfa and their dog with a big circle painted around its eye. And what was the name of Alfalfa's girlfriend?"

"Darla. I got this idea to take a gang of wild kids and have them running around in a studio like this, getting into all kinds of trouble. But I got the same problem as you do, no place to work," Ray said as he threw his wadded-up napkin on his plate.

"I'm getting by working on my story some nights in that dingy coffee shop on Wilshire, but I'm not making a lot of progress." Stephan wasn't too enthusiastic because he was tired today from a late night the evening before, which added to his sense of depression. He reached for his plate and mopped up the remnants of his rice and beans with a soggy corn tortilla, quickly popping it in his mouth before it collapsed.

There had been a concert the night before at a club called The Blue Moon Saloon by the beach in Venice that Stephan had gone to with Greg and a fellow crewmember. They had hung out after the show, partying with the band called Jiva, who had recently moved to LA, seeking their fame and fortune. They had all hit it off well, Stephan and

Greg boogying to the funky rock tunes with some local ladies on the sawdust-covered floor. Later, they bought a tape from the manager who also ran the soundboard that led to a few rounds of beers with the band members. The lack of sleep and overabundance of alcohol had flattened Stephan, who was used to early nights and the rare drink in his pursuit of a healthy lifestyle.

Ray pointed across the canteen to a slightly paunchy man wearing a suit, who looked to Stephan like he was in his thirties, addressing a table full of people from the studio. Ray said, "That guy over there would be a good source of career counseling for you."

The man's suit had eye-popping plaid squares with lapels as broad as airplane wings and he was speaking with a fast-talking style that made it look like he was working a hustle on the crowd. Stephan had noticed him around a couple of times at lunch and assumed he might have been managing the studio.

"The guy's name is Roscoe Malone, astrologer to the stars. He's got a fancy office in one of the buildings just inside the gates."

"Maybe getting my chart done could give me some clues on how to move forward."

Ray took Stephan over and proceeded to introduce them. Malone was friendly and shook hands but had a superior air. Stephan noticed that even though there was a projected air of aristocracy, Malone was one of those people that could make a two-thousand-dollar Italian suit look like it was off the rack at a Wal-Mart. Dressed in his one-hundred-dollar suit from a men's discount shop,

Malone could have passed for a mid-market used-car salesman. Stephan was respectful and ended up making an appointment for a counseling session. He knew from experience that astrological advice from a so-called expert could be just as accurate as the Sidney Omarr column in the daily paper but thought any extra insight could be useful at this point. Stephan had some money saved and even though the reading was relatively expensive thought it was a good investment.

He was glad for the opportunity to get some advice on his situation as he and the crew were off again to the hot end of the San Fernando Valley to pick up more heavy, oversized backdrops in a sauna-hot warehouse that amplified the already hundred-plus heat. Some would call a job in the film industry heaven, but this was as close to hell as Stephan could imagine, from the debilitating heat all the way down to the poisonous food in the canteen. He hoped the astrologer could help him find a ticket out of there, although an inner sense made him guess that this was only purgatory and the real fun was about to begin.

7

PRODUCERS STUDIO

Roscoe Malone's eclectic business style reflected the independent nature of the founders of the studio where his offices were housed. Producers Studio was a relic from the glory days of 1920s Hollywood, when Charlie Chaplin, Douglas Fairbanks and a couple of their acting pals had started their own production company to free themselves from the studio system that owned actors. They pooled their resources and founded their own studio on a chunk of land in Hollywood across the street from one of their former employers.

Their studio had long ago faded into obscurity after the actors drifted back to work with the majors. They had followed the evolutionary cycles of Hollywood, when the studio bosses' power was replaced by the influence of agents who took to packaging deals with their clients as the centerpiece. The lot remained as an independent production center for TV shows and music videos on the low end of the Hollywood food chain.

The studio's entry was built in a ten-foot tall chain-link fence that wasn't quite as elegant as the white Moroccan-style arched gates of Paramount that faced them on the other side of Melrose. A modest show of security was in place, with a rent-a-cop in a small security hut on busy days or, more typically, one of the studio secretaries in the administrative office facing the gate checking names on a daily list of approved visitors.

Stephan entered the studio one muggy morning when the coastal fog still hid the Hollywood sign, and was ignored by the studio staff who couldn't be bothered to get up from their coffee to check him on the day's guest list. After a couple of weeks of working on the lot, he was a familiar face so was given a quick wave and didn't have to sign in. Stephan ambled along the Wild West plank walkway that fronted the building across from a huge soundstage, his footsteps echoing on the wooden slats. He peered into grime-covered windows, occasionally spotting some activity going on. The first two offices past the gate had notepaper with company names written on them in big letters taped inside the window, indicating a production in progress. The remaining five or six offices on the way to the stairs to the second floor were furnished but empty. Across the driveway one tall soundstage had its massive doors open revealing a set that looked like a 1950s nightclub with the crew scurrying around moving equipment for the next scene. The stage next door was quiet for the moment but in the evenings, Frank Zappa could be heard rehearsing with his band.

The upstairs hallway in the old studio building was dusty and dimly lit, with no visible signs of life. The worn-out linoleum flooring that simulated green marble was a peeling obstacle course of holes with curling edges. This abandoned office block was one of several in the studio complex and could have been a long-forgotten film set waiting to be dusted off and repopulated with a crew and actors. Ghost offices contained empty desks and filing cabinets of departed executives from the good old days; it looked like a neutron bomb had hit, leaving the infrastructure while vaporizing the inhabitants.

A distant sound of typing could be heard ahead as Stephan searched for the famous astrologer, with only the faint light from smudged windows along the hall to illuminate the way. Stephan passed a door where the sound of typing now sounded maniacal; however, there was no sign to indicate who the occupant was, so he moved on. The next door had a tall row of brass nameplates attached to the doorframe. The signs read from top to bottom: Roscoe Malone Consulting Astrology, Globall Corporation, Great Impressions Publishing, Fourth Dimension Enterprises.

The door was ajar, and someone was talking on a phone on the other side, so Stephan tapped quietly and pushed it opened. Malone sat behind a huge desk piled high with books, brass astronomical instruments and stacks of papers. Underneath the desk's glass top were various official-looking documents and antique maps while shelves around the desk were filled with curios, like carved animal figures, antique letter scales and microscopes. Malone waved him in, and Stephan nodded a hello while observing all the odds and ends piled up in every free space.

Malone looked like a carnival barker in a white shirt and suit vest with the only thing missing being a garter on one sleeve. His dark hair was cut short in the front but reached over the collar of his shirt in the back like a Prince Valiant look. He was working some kind of spiel on the phone, talking up one of his businesses, so Stephan studied the endless rows of framed black-and-white photos of Malone's clients that filled all the walls in a mosaic of a captured audience. Most were autographed with some sort of dedication, but Stephan didn't recognize anyone even though a lot of the standard audition pictures had the person's name and contact information printed cleanly across the bottom. Some referenced defunct TV shows and Stephan willed himself to believe that one actor was vaguely familiar.

A couple of would-be actresses gave their best side to the camera to look cute in their dramatic poses. Each sheet typically had one main photo and two smaller ones, with some personal data and credits on the bottom. The large picture was usually an elegant pose, with styled hair and evening gown and the other two would be more fun, to show the actress's range and diversity.

The one Stephan liked best was a photo of a born-again blond in a low-cut cocktail dress with her hair piled up as the main image that contrasted with the same lady in pigtails and bib overalls sitting on a rail fence. The third photo depicted her in a 1950s bobby-soxer costume with waved hair, pushing her skirt down between her knees like a precocious high-school student sitting on the Senior Bench. The smile was a bit naughty as if to suggest she could be a bad girl when required. Stephan wondered about copying down the phone number, but then thought better of it as every other guy passing through the office would have had the same idea.

Malone beckoned him to sit down in a faded red leather armchair as he finished his pitch with a flourish and hung up.

"Excuse the mess." Malone waved one hand dismissively in the general direction of the most clutter. "Looks like that property manager has beat you down with all those sets to move around," he said sympathetically.

"Indeed. It's the usual circus on the soundstage," Stephan answered in an upbeat tone glad for some sympathy from someone who knew the game.

Malone asked how the film work was going in the heat and if the production was wrapping up. Stephan explained the shots were taking longer because the actors kept falling down due to a shaky stage. Malone's eyes lit up at the mention of an accident and after explaining that fixing the stage would save money considering all the people standing around he also mentioned in a quieter voice that it would also avoid any possible lawsuits. There were no apologies from Malone over the appearance of the offices. The regal air he projected was worthy of a CEO or studio head and his role was perpetuated so believingly Stephan was initially impressed.

"Okay, so let's get down to the basics. Can you tell me exactly where and what time you were born?" Malone asked.

The first part of the consulting session was a background description of the various influences that shaped Stephan's life and the resulting tendencies. A few crosschecks such as to the nature of his family life allowed for some dialogue back and forth. Malone orated on the more praiseworthy traits and shifted to a personal tone for the possible negative issues to deal with.

Stephan's life had been relatively uneventful as a child of the California suburbs with a father who was an engineer at a defense contractor and a housewife mother tending to household duties for him and his two sisters. His parents were British and brought some of the old-world culture to the other side of the pond as well as a touch of a bohemian lifestyle. His mother painted landscapes, which adorned the family living room and wrote short stories that never got published, so was the dreamier, creative influence on Stephan in his early years that balanced the more rational side of his father's nuts-and-bolts approach to life. But both parents loved music, which meant show tunes from their past and an old piano in the dining room assured the house was always filled with songs. The friends he had in high school were mostly musicians or artists who exposed him to the Sixties idealism that their older brothers and sisters had lived and tried to keep alive. Some of the loose-knit suburban clan he ran around with had been reading books on yoga and Eastern philosophy and the spirit of the themes hooked him so that he would read every book he could on the subject in the local library and hitchhiking to the Los Gatos old town area to find new ideas in the funky bookstore catering to counterculture types.

A couple of brothers from high school formed a band with some recent graduates and he hung out at their apartment learning how to drink beer and separate the seeds from the stems in a shoe box lid. They followed bands like the Doobie and Allman Brothers and anything that came from England. At the same time another group of friends from high school had evolved their blues band in a jazz direction, and while the young lady thought she was the next Billie Holiday her Latino boyfriend perfected his John Coltrane sax styling.

Stephan met James at a party for employees at Atari, an electronic games company where the older brother of a high-school friend was working on an assembly line. Stephan and James became instant friends as connoisseurs of music and being fellow seekers of truth. They met in local parks or at each other's homes to exchange their latest findings while James continued to work with Grok, building on their successful dynamic of selling blue boxes by looking at commercial (and legal) projects. Meanwhile Stephan had started going to college in Berkeley studying English and journalism.

Malone had commented that Stephan's interest in spiritual subjects was normal for someone with the planetary configurations and aspects his birth chart indicated. And with a Libra ascendant, the scales, as a primary influence it was natural for him to seek balance and harmony. Malone had a small cassette recorder running and changed the tape over towards the end of the analysis. The next part was what people paid this soothsayer a hundred bucks an hour for – the progressions. This is where Malone would progress the sky map forward to show what influences would be present in the future, usually in a three- and six-month time frame. Until now Malone had been fairly accurate, but then any sharpie looking Stephan over and having a chat with him could accurately guess some general tendencies.

This was Hollywood, and any psychic, astrologer or person who reads the lumps on a head to tell the future could always find willing victims among the insecure hopefuls, as well as those who tenuously held on to their position as a star, having arrived there with no clue how and also having no idea why their popularity was sustained. If they could unlock the key to that conundrum, fame and fortune would be everlasting, which was the modest wish of these humble show folks.

The tendencies were clear – with Jupiter in the ninth house, squared with Saturn, the communications field was a natural avenue for career possibilities. Just looking at Stephan getting a journalism degree and working on writing projects at such an early age, wasn't that proof enough of a calling in mass communications?

The last bit of advice Malone introduced was to suggest Stephan acquire an emerald as soon as possible to enhance the better Jupiter tendencies in his chart, as the color green would amplify the planet's beneficial tendencies. Having similar influences, Malone sported a big chunk of an emerald crystal in a large gold ring adorned with some mystical symbols. The chart notes and label on the cassette were also written with a green Flair felt-tip pen, as according to Malone, green being the color of money meant that like attracted like. Malone always wore at least one item of clothing in green and had even covered his office shelves with green felt. Stephan understood the concept in principle but knew it more from the Hindu idea of karma where actions attracted like actions, so seeing it used as a cash machine struck him a bit odd.

Finishing with a flourish, Malone said all signs looked good for a healthy, successful future, full of creative accomplishments, willing women and that will be fifty bucks please. Stephan gladly accepted, reassured his destiny was now clear and happy to pay half the usual rate not knowing why he got a discount, although that was soon to become clear. Malone had stood up and hooked his thumbs in his belt and looking at Stephan with an expression of trust and appreciation said, "Look, I've got a business proposition that might interest you. And if you take me up on the offer I could waive the fee for today's session." The formal part of the session was officially over and they could chat now as mere mortals again, acquaintances on their way to becoming friends.

Malone was expanding his domain of mail-order companies, wholesale and publishing businesses and needed to ramp up staff and hire his first employee. Malone had a series of part-time secretaries that had helped out in various capacities, but with an aggressive growth plan, most likely inspired by beneficial star sign configurations, the time to build up real staff to ride the auspicious planetary aspects was now.

The Malone Empire stretched across several offices, half of which were squatter status. The studio management didn't care about this upstairs wing as it was generally too broken-down to rent any of the space, except to the occasional production companies who needed temporary offices for a few months. It had been over a year since the last neighbors pulled up their stakes. The only other tenant on the floor was a TV screenwriter in the next office who had sold one script to a cop show a year ago, and struggled to find the winning formula to sell a second one.

Malone started to pitch Stephan on the idea of working for him in his publishing business. "This is a rare opportunity to get in on the ground floor and more important is that you can build on the key strengths that are clearly indicated in your chart – communications, specifically publishing. You can learn the finer side of management and ultimately be in charge of your own enterprise, which will give you time to do what you really want. Look, I'll be honest, the pay is low but you have a chance to be a part of something, create a business from scratch. What do you say?"

"Well, I'm grateful you would consider me to be part of your operations. It sounds too good to be true." Stephan thought the reading had seemed a bit contrived and Malone's various businesses smelled a bit shady but if he could escape the manual labor while he got better integrated into the local scene it was an interesting option to consider. Also, understanding the dynamics of the publishing business could be a bonus. He would insist on getting paid in cash. "Sounds intriguing. The printed word has always attracted me, so it would complement my writing efforts."

"That's right, Saturn in Libra transiting the 7th house opposite Uranus – a natural." Malone held up the chart as confirmation. "I take that as an affirmative," he said in a gruff military tone and Stephan wasn't sure it was meant to be ironic or natural speech. "Great, welcome on board."

If James could start a computer company and Greasy

his own garage, Stephan thought maybe it was time for him to get into his own business. And as Stephan had been freelancing articles for small magazines during his college days, publishing seemed a natural extension of his creative talents.

Stephan's acceptance of the offer was rewarded with a lunch invite. Stephan felt conspicuous going to a restaurant in his cowboy shirt, bell-bottom jeans and boots compared to Malone's suit and tie, but he assured himself this was Hollywood, so anything goes.

They went out the studio gates and across Melrose to the parking lot by Paramount's south entrance where a small seven-stool Mexican café was located next to the little office that managed the parking spaces. Some crew from the studio were there and a couple of guys who looked more like directors or producers ate at a corner table. Malone and Stephan sat at the counter and loaded up on enchiladas and Pepsi with a couple of free refills from the friendly señorita behind the counter who took to flirting with Stephan in response to his friendly manner.

After Malone scanned the sports page of an abandoned *LA Times* they got down to basics. Stephan's first assignment would be the production of Malone's flagship publication – the *Second Annual Star Sign Calendar and Celestial Almanac – The Most Informative Calendar in the World* (according to the Malone Book of World Records). Back at the office, Stephan studied the mock-up of the upcoming edition with this year's dedication on the front cover made to a friend of Malone's who was heir to the largest muffler franchise in Southern California. Each day on the calendar was filled in with text giving vital information and historical news. Not only were there good haircut days, bad baking days, days not to sign contracts (Mercury in retrograde), buy clothes (Moon in Gemini) but also the best days to garden (first two quarters following the new Moon) and go to the bank. The rest of each day was filled in with planetary aspects, historical trivia, witty aphorisms, notable birthdays, practical advice and inside jokes for friends and clients. Stephan was dubious as to the accuracy and wondered if tossing a coin or consulting the Chinese oracle called the *I Ching* would be more precise.

The production was pretty straightforward, involving not much more than a large art pad three feet wide and two feet tall and a drafting table stolen from an abandoned office. A jar full of green felt-tip pens and ample bottles of white typewriter correction fluid were the tools of creation. The large pages would have a calendar grid and numbers for each day drawn on them, with the remaining task of filling in the details left up to Malone and now Stephan as his new editor, researcher, publisher, marketing executive and production slave.

Stephan started the next week, and although the pay wasn't great it beat flipping burgers at a grease pit or hauling around endless piles of film equipment and props. But soon, in spite of the grandiose promises, Stephan still needed to do some of the production assistant manual labor to meet the rent. Stephan persisted. He could see how Malone worked with suppliers and customers with a no-nonsense approach that appeared organized and done with a drive to really build something. Perhaps the guy was really going to create the next mega-corporation and he could be a part of it. If nothing else, the business world was a new experience for Stephan providing a balance to his artistic leanings and making his writing more disciplined.

Greasy initially opposed the arrangement, as it meant his friend would be moving on from his sphere of influence. Greg considered himself Stephan's mentor, being an old friend and several years senior. And having also had his chart done by Malone, he was suspect of Malone's seriousness. Nothing tangible he could name, just an intuitive sense of something that bordered on charlatanism. He tried to warn Stephan one night in the garage.

"I know he may be a bit dodgy as an astrologer but some of his analysis makes sense," Stephan said. He was making a half-hearted attempt to defend Malone from where he was perched on an old bar stool by a grungy workbench full of old car parts he was afraid to touch for fear of getting coated with grease.

"Come on – the guy is a master of telling people what they want to hear. It doesn't take a genius to know you're not happy busting your backside." Greg was pacing the room, fiddling here and there with tools and scattered elements from motors.

"Sure, but he also offered me a step towards escaping the slave job."

"Yeah – by offering you another slave job. Besides, everyone I talk to says he's only one step ahead of the law which means you could get into trouble."

"Maybe you're right. But working for him isn't the same as being a partner."

"What happened to our plan to open a yoga center? We're not going to stay in LA forever – just long enough for the heat to die down up north. Then we can get back to our dream of really helping people." Greg picked up his socket wrench and started to wipe it with a rag.

Stephan replied sagely, "My friend, you seem to forget James told us last week that you are still on everyone's shit list and we know that families can carry a grudge for a long time."

"Come on, you're going to throw all your spiritual studies to the wind for some hustler's business plans?" Greg replaced the wrench and picked up a large screwdriver he started to wipe down.

"Whoa – slow down a second. I'm never going to lose that connection to what is valuable and if I want to share my writing with the public it's good to know how to promote it." Stephan was quiet for a second staring out the open garage door at the backyard as he reflected on his priorities. He felt like the world was spinning faster and faster and that he would have to modernize his outlook to keep pace with the changing times.

Greg broke his reverie. "Up north we had us a good little scene going and you were much more focused. Or, I should say, you had more time for your work. Here it's like we're both caught up in a whirlwind. I'm trying to look out for you so you don't get seduced by the illusion."

"Thanks, man. I'll keep my eyes open. But you should also keep the faith, brother. Before we left, your yoga classes were more a place to find your latest lover than a serious house of healing."

"Helping people takes on all forms, so don't judge someone else's approach," Greg said with a sly wink tossing the rag he had been holding in Stephan's direction where it landed on the workbench.

Late-nighters in the office were common towards the calendar's publication deadline, to finish the content and allow time for printing and distribution in the fall season. Entertainment was a never-ending stream of groupies, B-girl starlets, loud drinkers, film riffraff and hangers-on who would float in and out until the wee hours. They would call from the payphone outside the gates and Stephan would have to run down to let them in. The gate was closed at night with a chain and combination lock to which Malone always managed to find someone to tell him the weekly combination, even though it was against the studio rules.

The loud parties would be supplemented by an old record player, where a stack of records on the spindle would fall one by one to the turntable. Malone wasn't a music connoisseur, so the same stack always got lifted back in place with the identical songs repeated all night. It was like the drums on a galley ship – beating the rhythm to drive the workers.

It wouldn't be unusual for Malone to disappear at 2 a.m. with some fluffy-haired blond with silicon enhancements, leaving Stephan to lock up. Stephan worked away in the back room like an indentured servant while Malone entertained his public as part of his persona of corporate head and chief executive officer.

Once the pages were printed and bound with a green

binding they were mailed to clients from Malone's huge list of astrological victims, friends and acquaintances. A few local bookshops stocked the calendar and Stephan went knocking on doors to sell more. There were several big bookstores by Hollywood and Vine that were customers and the main one on the corner that had a large metaphysical section featured a copy of the calendar prominently in its main window. Stephan managed to locate a statewide distributor who put the calendar in their catalog and a couple of small ads were placed in different astrological and New Age health publications to generate more orders. The efforts paid off and the calendar would have its biggest year ever with orders from the ads coming from as far away as New York.

Other work for Great Impressions Publishing started to drift in. Using some embossed business cards with his name and title on them, Stephan was able to impress a non-profit organization enough to allow him to manage the production of a monthly newsletter. It was a break from searching the stars and balanced the seasonality of the calendar with a more regular monthly income.

A couple more clients appeared including LA's first Spanish language TV station that needed someone to manage an in-house publication. This job required great diplomacy, as Stephan had to perpetually fight off the advances of the station manager. She was the female equivalent of the hard driving lady exec that Faye Dunaway portrayed in the film *Network*, whose sexual frankness and forceful attitude earned her an Oscar.

The *Star Sign Calendar* was the flagship publication,

but to bolster the company's catalog, Malone was planning a few additional projects that included his own get-rich-quick book. He fancied himself a modern-day Ben Franklin, spinning practical homilies in the calendar like 'a penny saved is a penny earned' (although Stephan would eventually wonder if 'a penny stolen is a penny found' were more the case) and then using some of these themes as the basis of his book.

Some of the other titles that were getting solicited from the respective authorities in their subject area included *How To Play the Ponies – A Track Insider's Foolproof Winning System*', '*Tax Shelters Of The Rich And Famous*' and '*Tantric Massage – What The Kama Sutra Left Out*'. The last title intrigued Stephan, as he looked forward to meeting the mystic mama of the potential bestseller and talking with her about the yogic wisdom and human potential elements of her area of practice.

Mail order and multi-level marketing were Malone's vision of an independent business and his Fourth Dimension Enterprises sold everything from imitation leather shoes to pyramids for razors so they would never need sharpening. And to complete the range of activities Malone was also approaching possible 'investors' for buying Mexican oil futures, where he had a contact with a firm south of the border sure to strike it rich on their claims in the Gulf of Mexico. The Arab oil embargo of 1973 was a recent memory of long lines forming at the gas pumps that made investors think of oil as a sure bet. Malone's eternal optimism and motto of 'make it big' meant Stephan was never sure if the deal was an elaborate scam and possibly illegal or else Malone's ticket to millions that would let him light fat Havana cigars with hundred-dollar bills.

Malone's personal history was the stuff of legends Stephan patched together from a few inadvertent comments from Malone, clues from the TV screenwriter next door, plus details some friends provided, so that a picture began to emerge. Malone had attended UCLA for four years, which was a placeholder for an undecided life, and he ended up with a degree in history. His father was a lawyer in Orange County, with a second career gambling on horse races, so as a child Malone was exposed to the well-to-do hanging around at Hollywood Park during racing season.

Following graduation, Malone had done a family-sponsored sabbatical in England to study culture and history but was mostly lending expertise on antique purchases for rich tourists, all for a commission of course, using his knowledge of English history to embellish his scanty expertise with antiques. Malone had no fear of moneyed individuals, having drank and joked with Southern California's finest at the races. He could talk a good story, especially after an afternoon of entertaining in a pub.

With his cash reserves, Malone was able on his return to LA to fund his office set-up and, with business deals besides his usual operations, could maintain a positive cash flow. There were mysterious visitors in three-piece suits who would drop by after dark. Their discussions were held out of earshot as well as those with the studio management and freelance producers all of whom maintained small bungalows in a corner of the lot. Malone hinted at celebrated restaurant meetings or get-togethers in stately homes like the Getty mansion in Malibu; Stephan never really understood the scope or extent of Malone's arrangements.

After several months Stephan was starting to wonder about the longevity of the set-up and was considering other options. And yet the cachet of working for a media and publishing company in LA was seductive. Word of his ability to acquire projects and publish got around his circle of friends so that everyone from mad poets on Venice Beach to free-spirited ladies with children's classics they had written for their child approached him.

He liked walking across Melrose to the modern offices of the Spanish TV station humming with activity. There was a feeling of power he got from presenting projects in a stylish meeting room for the consideration of the marketing manager and other senior staff while the station manager flirted from a sofa in the corner adjusting her miniskirt so he could glimpse flashes of her electric red panties while he was making his pitch. Going back to his offices was a study in contrasts as the TV station was completely public and above-board while Malone's affairs had the air of some kind of a scam. Sometimes he felt he was investing his energy in the wrong direction but this impression was balanced by the quasi-artistic nature of his business that was truer to his roots.

8

ART FOR ARTISTS' SAKE

Villa Montalvo was a stately Italian mansion hidden in the foothills above Saratoga, perched on a tree-lined ridge like an unexpected mirage. Crowning a majestic green lawn, the villa was surrounded by a hundred acres scattered with exotic Mediterranean plants. It was an oasis of European sophistication with its main focus on nurturing artists of all disciplines, from classical music to painting. The halls of the main house were lined with rare art, and the main reception area welcomed guests with a hushed air of sophistication in the midst of gilt furniture and marble floors.

The senator who donated the property to the city of Saratoga wanted it to be an 'Athens of the West', in the noble Renaissance tradition of fostering the arts through the sponsorship of well-to-do individuals and corporations. Dating back to when the center first opened in the 1930s, many cultural events had been held with influential writers, artists and performers; Villa Montalvo was the oldest artist community in the West.

Maria had received a scholarship that provided her with a workroom in one of the wings of Montalvo's main house, and allowed her to attend classes with various guest artists.

She had been painting in various formats since her early teens and had already seen her work featured in a couple of local galleries. She spent three days a week at the villa, with the remaining days at Stanford working on a degree in art history. While the schooling pleased her parents, they had hopes she would shift her major to a more academic subject or at least get a teaching degree.

Maria could breathe easier in her private studio, safely away from her close-knit, overbearing Italian family. Lately it was more her place of refuge to deal with the loss of her childhood friend, while struggling with her nascent romantic interest in somebody who was connected to the incident. And yet not wanting to let James go completely, she'd managed to return a few of his many calls. The contact had intensified the battle of the conflicting feelings of her strong attraction for him and the knowledge that a relationship with him would be, in the eyes of her family, seriously discouraged if not outrightly condemned due to the nature of his work and being considered an accessory to Tobias's death. While her intellect told her the best thing was not to get involved further, her heart whispered encouragement in her ear so that she couldn't quite let him go. Then too, part of her wondered if James could be some kind of opportunist chasing the first woman he liked at the party. And yet, she doubted his talk of being an artist was an act, sensing someone with a creative side, with a depth beyond just the world of electronics. But then what kind of person could he be to engage in such a reckless activity like a late-night race? As people are known by the company they keep, perhaps this was a clue to another side of James she had yet to see. Ultimately, she knew that Tobias's parents saw their son as a martyr, who died nobly, sacrificing his life in the cause of farmers' rights.

She had one confidant close-by with whom she could discuss her conflicted feelings – the family housekeeper. The lady was of Mexican descent and everyone called her Mamacita as she had been with the family for as long as anyone could remember, her real name lost in time. Mamacita had been Maria's nanny and surrogate mother since she was born and knew Maria better than her own parents. She had wisely recognized the spell of young love in Maria's moodiness after meeting James, following years of trying to explain the mysteries of romance and courtship to the young woman in hope that she'd find a suitable partner.

Two nights after the accident Maria had been in her bedroom making a feeble attempt at studying when Mamacita knocked quietly and entered. She went over to where Maria was sitting on a sofa and sat next to her and said she knew something was troubling her, more than just Tobias's death.

Nodding her head, Maria said, "It's true, Mamacita, and I'm so confused. Saturday night started out as the best day of my life – I met this wonderful man – and then it turned into the worst."

"We all are suffering, my little angel. It was such a shock for the whole family."

And then Maria explained James's connection to the accident. "What hurts is that somebody I felt an instant connection with, somebody I felt I could really love has turned out to be a reckless person," Maria said.

"You cannot blame one man for another's actions. That DiFilippo boy was always racing, so it could have been anyone challenging him."

"You're right, Mamacita, but my family don't want to see it that way."

"We are going to have to deal with that, sweetheart, if you think this man could be your love."

"Thank you." Maria leaned over and hugged Mamacita. "I don't really know this James person but we have such a lovely contact when we speak and I'm sure we could get to know each other better. He's so sensitive and understanding. Never mind his profession."

"Then, my dear, you must listen to your heart. Your emotions are swirling around like troubled water but once they settle down you will have more clarity and know if you want to see him again."

While Maria had most of her days filled with classes, James was in a crucial phase of his business that required his presence around the clock as new designs were finalized and translated into deliverable products. The new investors supported James's vision of one integrated device in a simple and elegant case rather than the motherboards screwed into a wooden frame with separate power supply and connectors that was the standard in the fledgling market. James's vision meant breaking new ground, not only in trying to build a plastic housing to his exact design and integrate all the electronics but also believing the public would respond favorably. It meant Grok had to step up and improve the operating system so the device could do more functions and support programs that were useful such as one based on a new idea called a spreadsheet. James knew 'The Spreadsheet' could be big, very big. But he was racing against time; his competition wasn't sleeping. His drive and demand for technical perfection kept the young company moving forward, and his presence was more decisive than the president recently installed by the new underwriting venture capital company. Since commercial decisions drove manufacturing schedules and product features, James, with his sense of vision, always felt he had to defend the integrity of the product, pushing for more time and space when he felt it was needed. He worried if he wasn't around fighting for his products that there could be a coup and he would be marginalized. Worse than that, his vision would be hijacked and transformed into something that wouldn't reach his idealistic goals. And with outside investors, he was obligated to prove his dream was something real.

Even though he was immersed in the business operations his thoughts kept going back to Maria, and at least three or four times a day he tried to call her. Mamacita would always answer the phone and, he imagined, reluctantly told him she wasn't available. Early on he'd asked if he should stop trying to call, and when Mamacita tersely answered, "Try again," he took that as encouragement to keep calling. Finally, several days after Mamacita's gruff encouragement he managed to reach Maria and had the first of several brief chats as he tried to build on the feelings of their first encounter and deal with the awkwardness of the race. The calls were short and James felt like he was treading water, not sure if he would sink or swim, but the fact they kept talking raised his hopes. On the third call she gave in to his 'won't take no for an answer' pleading and agreed to meet him at Montalvo.

Irrationally afraid that his beloved red-and-white VW bus with the wild company graphics might be spotted by somebody at the villa who knew Maria's family, he decided to fall back on his old standby of hitchhiking to the mansion from Saratoga. Dressed in his work uniform of a black T-shirt and faded jeans, he strolled through the gravel parking lot alongside the main building.

Montalvo was named after the Spanish writer who created the name 'California' to describe a rich island populated by Amazons, led by a queen named Califia. The Amazons flew around on griffins guarding the treasures of the land, and the hushed, museum-like mansion had sculpted griffins in the cornices of the larger rooms as symbols of the estate. As James navigated the hallways of framed paintings and small sculptures he located the studios in a wing of the main building. He wondered if the family would be guarding Maria with the same watchful eyes as the griffins. With his long hair and scruffy face, James felt conspicuous imagining that the matrons running Montalvo would want to stop him from contaminating the refined artists in residence. But his intensity and ease with words left them standing in his wake wondering if he was another resident genius artist they hadn't met before.

When he finally found Maria's workroom and gently knocked, James's heart was pounding so fiercely he thought it was going to explode. He feared a family watchdog would be standing guard to ward him away, or worse – that he would be met with rejection. Maria opened the door looking like a modern Renaissance artist in a red embroidered blouse, bell-bottom jeans hanging on for dear life to her slender hips, bare feet and paintbrush in one hand.

They looked at each other awkwardly for a moment and each broke into a smile. They shyly embraced with a quick peck on the lips when they pulled apart.

"Please come in," Maria said formally in a mock aristocratic accent, standing back and sweeping her arm in a gesture of welcome. She crossed to a low armchair facing a sofa and plonked herself down as James closed the door and came over to sit on the sofa. An easel stood in the corner with a work in progress, a colorful landscape with a corner of the villa visible on one side. There was an awkward moment trying to find where to start but James broke the silence first.

"I'm so, so sorry about Tobias. I know it must be a huge loss for your family. And I know because my friend was involved it's made everything really complicated."

"I'm glad you understand." Maria smiled bravely reflecting for a second on the memory. "It just all happened so fast. Him dying and…" She hesitated. "You."

"I hope you know there was no intent for harm," James said.

"There never is in those situations," Maria said. "Nothing good is ever going to come from people engaging in a high-risk activity like racing cars when they're drunk."

"You're right. Of course you're right. And I guess you know that Tobias was the only person who was drinking." James was carefully weighing his words because from her responses he could see that she didn't know what the cause of the race was. His feelings were churning because mentioning it could end the relationship before anything got started but he also knew he had to be completely open and honest with her.

"If you knew that, then you or your friends should have had the wisdom to stop the race."

"There was no way he would listen to a single word any of us would say, including his own friends. He wanted to race and show that he had the better car."

"Well, your friend could have refused to race and been called a coward or whatever. I hear he teaches yoga. Not a very enlightened behavior for a yoga teacher."

Maria was tearing up, ready to start crying. She wiped her eyes and spoke in a constricted voice. "But it's over now, we can't bring him back."

"I wish him peace. Wherever he is. And if I can say this, wish the end of suffering for his family," James said gently leaning towards Maria wanting to hold her.

Maria shook her head and took a deep breath to regain her composure. "It's not going to end anytime soon. It's so hard to imagine I'll never see him again. We grew up together, but we were never really that close. And you know how Italians are – family and friends are big."

"I can imagine. But you're okay – still able to paint?"

"Yeah, I'm getting along." Maria paused regaining her composure and turned to point to a large easel angled by the tall windows facing down the villa's lawn.

"That looks like one of Monet's paintings of the gardens in France. Where was that, Giverny?" James said.

She smiled. "I don't think it's fair to either Monet or me to make a comparison. It can limit my finding my own style."

Maria's painting was a highly colorful still life of an abstract landscape expressed in a soft dreamlike quality of small, delicate brush strokes. It reminded James of an Impressionistic style but yet not a copy of any one artist, rather a synthesis of styles expressed in her own special way which was true to that movement's techniques. The rows of bright red and blue flowers bordering the lawn were like bands of undulating color with individual bunches of flowers distinguishable as spots of intensity leading the eye upwards. They captured the play of light that gave depth and feeling to the images of nature further supporting the Impressionist styling. The hint of the villa's wide front steps shrouded under the low-hanging tree branches expressed as an angular form was a focal point that could be interpreted as a manmade structure contrasting the vibrant and wild nature that seemed to illustrate different worlds and their possible harmonious existence. The play of diffused light fragmented by the trees made small rounded shadows on the gravel walkway and corner of the lawn like dreamy reflections on water.

After complimenting her on the painting James explained how he had a secret side where he imagined himself as a poet. He liked the romantic image of spending all day in a small French café with a cigarette dangling from the corner of his mouth, scribbling with passion in a notebook while a coffee long gone cold sat ignored. This same artistic passion could be channeled into a vision to design something that not only had a practical humanitarian use but also was aesthetically pleasing.

While James was quiet for a moment and studied the painting, he could see that Maria sensed that he had something more to share.

"Tell me what's on your mind, Mister Mad Poet," Maria said.

James hesitated looking for the right words and feeling they were connecting on a deeper level knew she could sense he had something important to say, but he deflected the moment of truth. "I know this is going to sound strange, but in the world of technology the highest art is to create something unique, something no one else has done before or a new expression of an existing idea."

"Like a painter or musician creating a new form."

"Exactly. And when I see what you're doing and other friends of mine who are artists and musicians, I sometimes wonder if that really isn't my true calling in life."

"Maybe your devices are the art of the future. If you hold true to that belief and live your dream those ideals won't get lost," Maria said joining him on the sofa. James put his left arm over her shoulder, bending in to look at her. She leaned towards him and then they were kissing. But then, just as effortlessly as they began, Maria pushed him back.

"I feel so strange. On one hand I feel as though this is so right, but then I keep thinking about how we came together."

"But we met up before your friend was in his race. We liked each other. It was real and true."

"Yeah, and I was also a bit drunk."

"Sometimes wine is a truth serum," James said.

"Oh, come on. That's ridiculous." She smiled knowing he was right. "Why don't we get out of here and go for a drive."

They locked up the studio and got in Maria's broken-down Fiat she drove with great pride where it was parked amidst some Mercedes and Jaguars. She explained how her father had offered her a long-term interest-free loan to buy a new Ford or even a newer Fiat but she turned down his offer, rather choosing to work one summer in an art supply store to earn enough money for her own car. She was proud to have the car as a symbol of her self-made freedom. She didn't care if it was rusting and had a faded paint job, looking worse than the helpers' cars parked in the family's driveway, it was hers to go wherever she wanted, free of any possible parental-imposed limitations.

They drove to Stevens Creek Reservoir, a large county park a short distance north along the coastal foothills. Further up the densely wooded valley they passed the dam forming the northern side of the small reservoir where some sunbathers were spread out across the sloping concrete wall. A large dump truck filled with gravel bore down on them and roared past, forcing them to quickly close their windows to avoid the trailing swarm of dust.

Maria took a smaller side road that wound deep into the wild foothills and half a mile along pulled into a small turnout under a group of oak trees. She knew a trail and they hiked hand in hand into the woods enjoying the silence and perfume of the sage and pine. In a clearing under some trees, Maria spread a blanket she had brought along from her car.

They sat awkwardly next to each other, and James offered Maria a drink from a bottle of water and some dates from a small plastic bag he retrieved from the old backpack he was carrying. He plucked a long-stemmed sprig of tall grass and started to chew the end like a farm boy. There was sense of expectation that was tempered by their both being a bit nervous that the incident with Tobias could spoil the intimacy. Safe in their private nest, the warm sun melted their resistance to experiencing the closeness they desired from when they first met.

James leaned over, kissing her bare shoulder. Maria held his head to hers with both arms, kissing James on the back of the neck. He looked up and met her mouth with a hunger only a sex-starved yogi could have. Maria had pulled up the back of James's T-shirt, tugging it out of his jeans. She put both her arms underneath, savoring the warmth of his body, reaching her hands almost to his shoulders.

She sighed deeply with an open mouth as the sensation of skin on skin aroused her. Maria's head momentarily leaned back as she breathed faster and more audibly. James, mimicking her actions, gently untied the peasant blouse where it was secured in the front and lifted it with great care over her head. Her firm breasts and dark nipples were soon covered by his hands that he only removed long enough for Maria to lift his shirt off. He bent to kiss her breasts and she gently fell backwards, lay back and ran her fingers through his hair. He was kissing her belly now with a hand on either breast, massaging the now slippery nipples, feeling their hardness grow. She pulled him onto her, feeling ready and he soon felt her wet silkiness envelope him.

James supported himself on his elbows to let Maria breathe but held her close. The incredible softness of her hips against his and the sweet smell of musk made him nibble on the back of her neck where her hairline began.

Afterwards they held each other, listening to the wind in the trees. Maria rolled over and pulled on her blouse before she retrieved her leather-bound sketchbook from her shoulder bag. She began to draw with some colored charcoal, outlining a stand of oak at the edge of their small clearing with the leaves turning golden brown in the early fall. "It's so beautiful here; the plants and trees all have such interesting formations and colors as if they are the embodiment of nature spirits."

"Nice sketch pad you got there," James said admiring the fine leather.

"I never go anywhere without it because you never know when inspiration will appear," Maria said leaning over and kissing James. "It was a gift from my aunt in southern Italy who I visited last summer. She's the same one that introduced me to the Tarot."

"Cool. She some kind of a gypsy?" James stroked the finely finished edge, feeling the smoothness of the leather and then continued the movement to her bare leg.

"Just a wise old lady. It's an old family tradition because the Tarot originated in Italy where it's called *tarocco* or *tarocchi*. She's actually a witch, like me," Maria said, waving her stick of charcoal like she was invoking a spell. "You better be careful."

"I like to take chances," James said wrestling her to the ground. She pushed him away playfully and went back to her sketching while he lay on his back watching the branches of the sheltering oak tree swaying in the wind.

James tried to keep his mind focused on the sweetness of the moment but his thoughts kept drifting back to the truth he had hidden from Maria that gnawed at him even more now that they had become so close. He felt trapped, because it was only a matter of time before it would come out. It was a classic case of paralysis by analysis. Thinking about it froze his actions and the longer he waited, the bigger the issue would be when it finally was revealed.

Perhaps it was this lingering guilt and the unexpected closeness to Maria that made him later wonder if it was the right thing to have said at that serene moment. James was more the thinker, so making sense of emotions didn't always yield the most optimal results. He looked at Maria who, while appearing content, seemed to be within in her own world.

"You look so into your drawing I don't want to break your flow but I wanted to be up front about something."

Maria looked over at him with an expectant smile, as if he would say something naughty. She adjusted her position, tucking her legs under so she could face him more directly. "You're going to tell me you're actually married with children?" They both laughed.

"I don't know really how to say this but I believe in total honesty and openness."

"Me too. It's what creates trust and brings us closer."

James hesitated a second, leaned towards her on one elbow and took a breath before taking the plunge. "The race with Tobias and my friend? It didn't start because of two car freaks showing off, it was because your friend didn't want me to see you anymore."

"What?" Maria had a shocked expression. "What are you saying – that someone died because you couldn't have a civilized discussion?"

"It's not that simple—"

"We're talking about someone dying!"

"Tobias followed me out of the club and wanted to fight me in the parking lot. He didn't like the type of business I'm in and as a consequence, me seeing you."

"Okay, I think I understand." Marias voice shifted to a no-nonsense businesslike tone. "You're saying this all happened because of me. You men are all so Neanderthal!" She rolled over angrily and grabbed her jeans, pulling them on hastily. "I think we should go now."

"Wait a second. I wanted to be honest and clear so there are no secrets or weirdness. I really like you. Now I'm starting to think it was a mistake telling you."

"I like you too and appreciate your honesty but I need some time to think. I'm sorry." Maria hastily packed her drawing materials.

"But we have something – a special magic," James said as he gathered his clothes.

"Time will tell. Can we go now?"

9

CITY OF ANGLES

Greg was moving, Greg was grooving, from the Hollywood Hills to Malibu's shores. Shaking and baking, as the hottest thing to hit town this side of a mouth-blistering jalapeño chili molten lava salsa, with the women willing and the nights steaming. Holistic-chiro-prana-tantra massages for the lithe bodies of wannabe actresses sweating musk, patchouli or Chanel No. 5 from every pore, as caressing hands stroked away tensions and gave rise to new sensations.

Like an ancient Hawaiian king regally poised on a longboard at Waikiki, Greasy managed to ride the wave of popularity, using his connections to a hot producer. He deftly maneuvered through intimate encounters, effortlessly handling every twist, turn and break, ultimately ending up dating a petite blond actress named Venus from a TV series Stephan had been working on the past few months. The family comedy called *Eight is Enough* was a story of a father and new bride raising a brood of smart-ass kids from the husband's first marriage. The eldest 'daughter' in the show was attracted to Greg's smooth-talking ways and Swedish massage treatments and they were often spotted cruising

Hollywood Boulevard in her Mercedes with 'VEGGIE' vanity plates while bouncing along to a blaring radio.

Venus had adopted a healthy lifestyle to preserve her looks and energy in the midst of a demanding career and clung to a positive attitude for self-preservation. At every party they were the natural center of attention that was half by plan, half by nature. In Sunset Strip clubs their wild dancing was a show that no one else could rival, even earning them mentions in the *Hollywood Reporter* gossip column. But like all Hollywood movies there was a big climatic scene that was followed by 'The End' with the credits scrolling by. The Greg and Venus Story dutifully followed this formula, as Venus needed someone who could better progress her career, so the film was over with no sequel in sight.

The break-up compounded a slow drift into disillusionment that started to be reflected in how Greg was performing at the garage. One night after a tune-up and servicing on a Mini Cooper, Greg took Stephan and a girl they knew from the band on a test drive with the sporty car along a twisty stretch of Mulholland Drive to show off the cornering. It was a thrill ride for the passengers and then returning to the city Greg let his attention wander. On a rain-slicked straightaway of Beverly Drive he lost control, bounced over a curb and onto someone's lawn, pulling out a sprinkler head in the process with a support strut. The car was intact and back at the garage Greg removed the bent support and hammered it back to its original shape. But even to an untrained eye the dings from the hammer and slight twist that couldn't be removed meant Bill would see the lack of interest that Greg was starting to show in his work. Greg could have ordered a replacement part but didn't think or care that Bill would notice as long as the car still ran perfectly. The chipped ceramic wheel was another clue to the rough ride.

Greg and Stephan were hanging out in the garage one night after dinner reviewing their life in So-Cal, Greg taking the lead as usual, kicked-back in a worn-out armchair that had been rescued on the way to a thrift shop.

"Did you get to see any stars today or were you just chatting with the stargazer about the Andromeda constellation?"

"If you call a B-list actor in a toupee a star then yes, I had my daily quota."

"Malone wears a hairpiece?" Greg said taking a shot at the astrologer.

"Get out of here – I was talking about the guy who played the funny sidekick in all the Doris Day movies," Stephan said.

"Sorry, it's just that everything else about the guy is fake so why not his hair."

"I'm still not too sure if he's as bad as you think." Stephan was defending his employment decision but at the same time a part of him knew Malone could turn out to be another Hollywood opportunist, a conclusion he hoped wouldn't be true.

Greg shifted the discussion to avoid a debate taking a sip from a plastic cup he had filled with beer from a stash he kept hidden due to the household rules. "Man, this whole town is one big show. Every moment is an audition and all you hear are lines some hack writer concocted, not the person's authentic feelings."

Knowing Greg was referring to his most recent relationship, Stephan said, "I thought you said Venus was just a fling. Sounds like you're a little bitter about what happened." He took a quick drink from his beer and carefully replaced it behind a carburetor in case someone from the house wandered by.

"Well, I guess I have to admit she did get under my skin. Thought for a while there we had the right combination to go the distance. Then – poof! I'm history. She pulled the rug out from under me to be sure."

Greg got up from the chair where it was positioned next to the workbench strewn with tools and auto parts and turned the radio off as it started playing Frampton's 'Show Me the Way'. He was cursing about hearing the song the thousandth time today, as it seemed to pop up every fifteen minutes no matter what station you listened to. Stephan agreed but he suspected Greg was more allergic to Elton's 'Don't Go Breaking My Heart' that had just finished and was an echo of his feelings towards Venus.

"You should have convinced Bill she was the hottest thing in town and to put her in one of his movies. They both would have thanked you. I could see you doing a producer gig."

"Ain't my scene, brother. Kissing ass and talking shit is for people without a soul. No sir, I'm not cut out to be a player in this town."

"You could support those stressed-out people. Venus could network you with a lot of her friends for private yoga classes and massage treatments.”

“I would just be her girlfriends’ toy boy and one more nobody trying to find an angle to shake down the stars. At least I was building up something in Santa Cruz that was respected for what it is, not who I last slept with.”

“This city isn’t just about showbiz. There are millions of people who live here who have normal lives.” Stephan put his hand in a small pool of oil while reaching for his beer and looked around for a rag.

“Other than you and our roommates I’m still looking for some genuine people with a real life going on.”

“Jiva?” Stephan said as he wiped his hand on a grimy rag that may have put more grease on his hand than it removed.

“Okay, those guys are cool but other than that ain’t a lot of authentic folks to be found.”

Stephan knew that LA had its share of fun and games, but for Greg to make his unique high-profile imprint on it would be impossible. Greasy couldn’t control his fate as he felt he could back in Santa Cruz, but that option was for the moment still closed to him. James had relayed an update from Maria a couple of days earlier that Tobias’s father was still scouting the streets for Greg with revenge in his eyes. Greg became a restless soul while the road slowly beckoned. Compounding this restlessness, Greg had confessed to Stephan a couple of times he still felt culpable for his role in the death of Tobias and even all the distractions a Southern California lifestyle offered could not erase the deeply rooted guilt that lingered.

The comments would reawaken Stephan’s own sense of complicity in what happened and he’d chastise himself for suggesting a race, especially since one of the drivers was obviously drunk. He tried to rationalize his participation, telling himself he hadn't suggested the race should take place the same night. The end result of his circular worrying was the effect on his writing. The story took longer and longer to compose, and he felt he was ignoring his duty to the silent baba, generating guilt on a second front.

The rules in this town rewarded those who could get the next big deal for a starring role or a record contract, providing limos and willing groupies by the dozen. Greg had neither ambition nor talent in either of those directions. He had to face the daily reminder from every encounter with each waiter, waitress, bagboy and receptionist who wanted to be a star and had moved to this city of dreams to try and realize their goal, looking out with eyes asking if you knew someone who could get them their first deal.

The two of them discussed how the town was the perfect representation of maya – illusion – nothing was as it appeared. Everything from fake movie sets to people who talk so much bullshit you don't know if they're acting or real. And only a few of them who arrived at that holy grail of celebrity would look back and wonder what life was all about. They find their same problems still exist even when they have fame and riches. Most of them clinging to the life their publicist created, wanting it to be true out of lack of originality, sacrificed to portray a dream image. You don't know if your friends like you because of what you have or who you really are, and nobody is real. Don't look the part? A plastic surgeon is waiting to make your nose the right shape to get that film role. Boobs too small? No problem, get a little boost and maybe some liposuction on those cottage cheese thighs while you're at it. Capped teeth and dyed hair were the minimum adjustments to improve your image. You think you're scoring with the babe of the century but she's all put together. You get close and dark roots are showing and there's a perpetual grin from the stretched skin of a nip and tuck.

They agreed it must be sad to be recognized by most of the planet without even knowing who you really are inside. Those people feel the emptiest because if you have everything and still don't have happiness what are you going to do? Everyone's looking at you like you have it all but you see that it's really no different. You still have to put your pants on one leg at a time no matter how rich or famous you are. Plus, you can't cheat the Grim Reaper when he's knocking on your door. That's when the show folks start looking for another source of contentment. Drugs and alcohol are the obvious choices and therapy and encounter groups only provide a Band-Aid to their uncertainty. Curing the symptom, not the disease.

"Their whole world is just another Hollywood set but when the lights of reality are turned up they see it's only a movie," Stephan said.

"With all these insecure mega-egos you'd think we could cash in somewhere. I could trade my Levi's for an Armani suit and talk with a resonate voice about good vibrations," Greg said. "We could do an *est* style human potential thing – instead of Erhard Seminars Training we could do Greg's Enlightenment Training and Inner Therapy – GET IT."

Stephan laughed and finished his beer. "That guy's

making tons of money but I know you'd soon feel like a sellout telling people what they already know," Stephan said. "I guess we both still have some shit to sort out before we can think about teaching anyone."

"Right on, bro."

"There's this one beautiful phrase the silent baba told us: No one can make heaven on earth until he has made heaven inside himself first. It's like holding a candle in the dark which is not lit and telling others 'follow me'," Stephan said.

"I like that. At least we have the chance to remember a few breaths and be mindful of the moment," Greg said as he poured the last of the can of beer into his cup.

"That's one thing that can remind us of our focus – except for looking at your ugly face," Stephan teased.

Greg adopted the voice of a playful swami. "But, my child, if I were to possess a hound with your countenance, I would shave its ass and make him walk backwards. Much more pleasant for the eyes."

The wheel of life rolled on and Bill bought a Maserati and decided a more specialist mechanic would be required. Because the new love of his life would be housed at his home, the second mechanic could work at Bill's place in Pacific Palisades, with a luxury setting to twist bolts and set the compression. Bill stopped by the garage late one morning to share the news. Tools were scattered across a narrow door balanced on two sawhorses that acted as a workbench and old tires and engine parts were stacked in the back corners. Greg was leaning over the engine compartment of a Mustang changing sparkplugs, up to his elbows in grease as usual so they skipped the traditional hand slapping.

"My man with the plan! Why you checking out the wheels when you should be making deals?" Greg said in a rhyming tone as he twisted a sparkplug into place.

"You're the man, brother. Looks like a fast car there." Bill walked around the end of the car peering in the engine compartment.

"The V8 is bigger than most production cars so can outrun the best of them."

"Maybe we'll get a chance to see that. Just bought a Maserati for my collection."

"Very cool – stylish and fast." Greg straightened up from where he was bent over the engine compartment and laid the wrench on the worktable. He knew from his tone that Bill wasn't here to talk shop. At least not in the way he usually did when checking on the various works in progress.

"And very temperamental and selective about who touches her – just like an Italian woman."

"You know I'll treat her fine like all my ladies," Greg said soul brother to soul brother.

"I know you would. Only thing is, it has twelve cylinders and requires special tools so I lined up a guy who knows these cars inside out." Bill looked at Greg and made a slight shrug of the shoulders to say it was nothing personal.

"That guy must cost as much as the car. Give me a little schooling and your Italian racecar will be the fastest set of wheels this side of Rome." Greg wiped his hands on a rag like he was getting ready for another project.

"It kinda needs attention now. The previous owner treated her like a whore."

"No respect. Hey, no problemo – I can look over the guy's shoulder and pick up a few tips."

"I wasn't planning on having it down here. I'm letting the guy use part of my garage in the Palisades." Bill was walking slowly back around the Mustang, still inspecting the engine.

"I guess a special lady needs a cool crib. Would sure like to see the sexy mama sometime and check out her curves."

"You know me, always happy to make an introduction."

"I'll be sure to wear some protection before lifting her hood, if you know what I mean."

Bill laughed. "Always the charmer."

Greg's comments covered up a wave of self-pity that washed over him as if he wasn't worthy of the trust or valued as a person of skill – support his ego needed at that moment. A part of Greg also knew Bill was justified in his decision and didn't want to get too much into the details of some of the rough emergency repair work he had done on Bill's Mini Cooper that he knew must have been noticed.

With an attitude looking for direction and growing tired of the confining house scene, Greasy took to hanging out late at night, occasionally with Stephan in tow. This was in spite of an unspoken code of righteous behavior the house maintained under Barry's watchful eye, that included abstinence from drugs or alcohol. Greasy and Stephan would slip out through the kitchen door to track down whatever party might be going on when everyone was in bed.

One night they were hanging out with an aspiring actor,

a cashier at a porno movie theater on Wilshire, who was the roommate of one of the production assistants Stephan had met working on a TV movie. Stephan was reluctant to visit the theater but Greg was telling him not to be so hung up on concepts, so in the spirit of exploration they headed out and got in free to watch *Behind the Green Door*. Stephan was both shocked at Marilyn Chambers servicing four guys at once as much as he was amazed at how someone could be so uninhibited. After the show, they went to the sleazy guy's apartment and partied with him, trying some Moroccan hash while he told his tales of trying to make it as an actor.

Stephan never saw the aspiring actor again after that night, but a week later Greg went alone to pay another visit. And among the assortment of party materials, the scraggly ticket taker produced some heroin that Greg sampled, sniffing a couple of lines.

Stephan was shocked when Greg told him about it the next evening in the garage. "What the hell are you doing? That stuff is so destructive. It'll ruin your body and turn you into an addict." He wanted to protect Greg, but ended up sounding like he was parroting the anti-drug films from high school that spouted a less educated view than held by those it was meant to instruct.

Greg defended the experiment. "Lighten up; it's not a big deal. Was just a taste, and you can see I'm not a junkie. In case you hadn't noticed, this is part of pure hedonistic LA living, brother." He stood up from the bar stool he had been perched on and improvised a couple of lines from a song by a group named America that was getting airplay on the radio. "I been through the desert in a Porsche with no name, it felt good to be out of the pain." He looked serious for a moment. "When the Rolling Stones were here a couple of years ago Keith Richards turned on so many LA rockers to heroin and they're all still cranking out songs. Look at me – I'm normal. Besides, one little toot isn't addictive."

"I'm sorry, but I feel like I've fucked-up again." Stephan turned away to look out the open garage door at the back of the house.

"What are you talking about?" Greg walked over to where Stephan was standing.

"First I suggest a race that screws up your life and now I've introduced you to heroin," Stephan said in a resigned tone looking at Greg.

"Don't give yourself so much credit. Quit trying to be such a saint all the time carrying the weight of the world on your shoulders. I made some choices I didn't have to. You can call it karma or stupidity but it is what it is."

"We're always having to make choices in life but I'd rather not be presenting you with bad ones to choose from."

"Why don't you consider it my education then? You're a wise tutor helping me see the value of my actions as I learn from life."

Some nights the two explorers would be in Echo Park, partying in an old Victorian house with Jiva. Greg had managed to become a part-time roadie when the band had weekend gigs out of town and not only drove the rental van but also fixed the band members' broken-down cars to support some starving artists. The house in Echo Park attracted a constant stream of visitors, so Greasy and

Stephan fit in with the crew and spent many a night listening to the musicians jamming, while partying with the groupies.

In spite of their best efforts to hide their nocturnal adventures, Barry figured out what was going on. One night after dinner he asked Greg and Stephan to join him in his room. Barry was sitting on the edge of a mattress on the floor while his guests lounged on some large pillows.

"You guys have been very cool giving free yoga classes for your roommates and some healing massages." Barry looked at Greg when he said the word 'massage' but without a benevolent look of gratitude. "And I know you're both dedicated to your path of self-improvement but lately I can see your focus has wandered."

"If you are referring to our late-night explorations of this fine city I can explain everything," Greg said sitting up straight. "We're like superheroes shining a light into the dark soul of this city with our elevated thinking."

"The only elevated situation I can see right now is you including in your excursions looking for a new home," Barry replied firmly.

"Wait a second. We may have made some mistakes but nobody's perfect. We can take this as a warning and calm down a little," Stephan said.

"Stephan, I would like to believe you. I've been in your shoes myself and I can see that you and Greg have some more living to do before entering into a more serious phase. What you two are doing is creating a bad vibe for the other people who live here." Barry folded his hands together in his lap as if to signal the discussion was over.

"Who says we're not serious? I can be so serious you'll

choke and turn to dust. It just ain't my style to express it. I can party my way from one end of this city to another and still keep my focus. It's all about intent," Greg said sitting forward to look at Barry eye to eye.

"That may be true but this house is for people who have moved on from that stage in life. I'm sorry, but you'll have to find another accommodation. I have my duty to the household. I'm truly sorry."

Stephan landed in West LA by the juncture of Bundy and Santa Monica Boulevard, in a derelict neighborhood of low-rent apartments. He wasn't too surprised to see halfway down the block some small houses where Mexicans worked on their lowriders in the front yard. Some of the members of Jiva who had relocated there had tipped him off to a vacancy so he soon had his own place to call home when he took over a small bungalow from a British film editor who was moving back east.

Greg moved in with his latest girlfriend he had met through the band, who was a slinky blond executive secretary with a small apartment in Hollywood. She was worldly and sophisticated compared to Greg but he was too much fun to let go. There were even the occasional hints after a few weeks that Greg may have been making an effort at domesticity that seemed to indicate a possible evolution.

Even with a loving lady and a stable environment, Greasy slowly prepared mentally for the return trek north. Having now also burned most of his bridges behind him in the south, he was hoping the bridges ahead had been repaired. Unfortunately, the calls he had made to Santa Cruz only reinforced the impression that he was far from forgotten and in fact, an unfriendly reception would be waiting if he reappeared. Greg had been a big brother to Stephan but as Stephan grew more independent with a widening horizon that was more influenced by Malone, Greg knew his capacity to mentor was also over. Their roles had become reversed and now it was Stephan looking after Greg, which further compounded the dynamic of their exile in Los Angeles.

At the same time, Stephan had been witnessing the slow disintegration of Greg and thought that a move north might revive Greg's more idealistic side; the City of Angels seemed to have sucked Greg's soul dry. It was a no-win situation: Greg was again slipping between temporary housing and making money fixing broken cars in a low-level garage who hired him after his job ended with Bill. And yet going back to Santa Cruz could be extremely risky.

Close to the Christmas holidays the two friends drove up to Sunset and went into the Rainbow Bar & Grill and found a place in a small booth on the side of the large main room, booming with rock music. A waitress who looked like she was a groupie on the last Eagles tour complete with skimpy tank top, denim miniskirt and cowboy boots, took their order.

"Is that Elton John?" Stephan asked as a short, round man with big glasses and electric blue suit came in with a friend and headed up the stairs to the members' area.

"In this town you never know who you'll bump into," Greg replied. They surveyed the other booths while the waitress served them and could see if they wanted to play the Hollywood game at this level they would need some trendy clothes and stylish haircuts.

"Well, if this ain't a show and a half I don't know what is," Greg said nodding towards the center of the bar laughing. In Kansas it would have been mistaken for a Halloween party with most people dressed in costumes like Woodstock-era hippies and hangers-on to the rock industry with billowy hair. There was one of everything, from faded band T-shirts and washed-out jeans (for both sexes) worn with everything from flashy sharkskin suits or khaki green military surplus jackets to Nashville-style outfits with piping on the lapels that looked like music notation. The women either wore short shorts with halter tops and no bra or painted-on jeans and billowy blouses that cost a fortune to look like cheap ethnic bazaar souvenirs.

"Free entertainment included in the price of admission," Stephan said raising his glass in a salute.

Greg returned Stephan's gesture, took a drink and got straight to the inevitable point of their meeting – his return to Santa Cruz. "I reckon the two of us could put on a real show for these folks if we set our minds to it but this scene sure ain't for us."

"It's fun to watch but I think everyone's posing. All these old burn-out roadies trying to score with young groupies on the strength of some band they once toured with," Stephan said nodding towards the bar.

"Sad indeed. Can't say I'm going to miss it." Greg was shaking his head like he had seen enough of this scene.

"You really are going to leave, aren't you?"

"I have to take the lesser of the two evils and at least the one waiting up north is one I'm ready for. No surprises.

Down here no way of telling what kind of mess I'll end up in." They both turned to watch a hot twenty-something in a short skirt and mile-high heels strut by, prowling for some attention which most of the males gladly provided.

"I'm still worried about Tobias's father, he can really mess things up for you," Stephan said with a concerned tone as he rested his arms on the table to hold his glass with both hands.

"I know, but I'll have to look the situation straight in the eye one day and waiting doesn't make it any easier." Greg studied the swishing miniskirt some more.

"Maybe you're right. I would love to go with you but I want to see how things will work out here. The band is using one of my poems for a song and Malone may be as shifty as the sand dunes in the Mojave but it's only a step."

"Just make sure you don't miss taking the next step. And maybe that will be heading back north." Greg looked at Stephan with a smile as if his crystal ball had shown him a future of love, peace and happiness.

"You know I have an open mind." They both laughed. "But it won't be the same around here when you're gone. You remember all those back cracks you used to give at Sodom and Gomorrah beach?" Stephan asked. The nude beach in Malibu had been their weekend hangout. There they could do their yogi routine of letting the salt water dry on their skin and draw out impurities or the nasal cleansing with the crystal-clear water, when they weren't making the rounds jiving with the different groups of weird Hollywood types that would hang there because it was a totally free environment. They interacted with everyone, supporting them at the level where they needed it like the confused film executive whose head was messed up after he screwed a hooker and then found out the she was a he.

Their Frisbee tossing was legendary for its precision, free-style catches and strategic flights to meet beach babes. Instructions like 'toss it a little more to the left' would result in the disc landing right on the cutest girl's towel. And compassion wasn't lacking when a drunken blond wandered over from Zuma Beach totally loaded and had lost her bikini top. Stephan had gallantly given her his Om T-shirt like a real gentleman but never heard from her again. And after a day of cavorting and cleansing Greg would drive the beach crew back to Hollywood via Malibu Canyon. There they would stop at a remote horse corral to shovel loads of manure into the back of the truck for one of the people's garden only to get coated with it when they hit the freeway with all the windows open.

"And you haven't even showered since then, have you?" Stephan said playfully. Greg laughed and tossed the coaster from under his beer at Stephan's head like a Frisbee.

10

GARDEN OF EDEN

Maria surprised James by calling him a couple of days after their meeting at Montalvo, a bit sad and a little in love. She apologized for retreating from what she came to realize was a heartfelt encounter for each of them and suggested they meet again to have a talk. Maria confessed to being torn between loyalty to her family and the feelings she had for him. She wanted to have a look at his office and share some time with him to understand his world better. Maria warned he shouldn't plan anything for the afternoon of her visit. James was ecstatic to hear from her and agreed, shifting meetings to free himself up for whatever she had in mind.

Maria rang the doorbell by the front door of the office complex in Cupertino that was set in the middle of blocks of mid-sized retail shops and car lots. After ringing about five times there was a buzz and a click releasing the door. She walked up an industrial staircase of wide cement steps and was greeted at the main door by a longhaired young man with large framed glasses, tie-dyed T-shirt and worn-out jeans. After a friendly greeting he took her through a labyrinth of cubicles where about thirty young men similar in appearance to her guide were either assembling machines or typing on keyboards in front of large TV-like monitors. The man led her towards some glass-paneled offices in the back of the room where James was working. Passing row after row of cubicles she caused a stir amongst the programmers and engineers who were used to an exclusive boy's club atmosphere. She was like a vision from their most favorite sci-fi film, a version of *Star Wars*' Princess Leia come to life with a pigtail replacing curled-up braids. The room echoed with clacking keys and distorted music from a set of speakers mounted in the corners of the room. A few of the employees who were close to James looked at her suspiciously, knowing she represented the farmers' interests which meant possible conflicts down the road. James's office was a glorified cubicle with walls and every available surface was piled high with printouts and manuals. He greeted her with a quick kiss, hastily clearing a chair for her to sit down on while apologizing for the mess.

"I don't think my dad would worry about you taking over this valley if he saw your office."

"Einstein said that chaos and clutter is a sign of genius, so go ahead and laugh."

"I would if I knew what I was laughing at. Is that one of your computer things?" she said pointing to a wood and metal box covered in wires and semi-conductors with a large TV screen next to it.

"This is going to change the world," James said proudly.

"If you say so. Looks more like a high-school science project."

James turned on the power and the green colored

screen lit up displaying some characters. He typed in some commands and the display changed to some swirling electronic patterns.

Maria watched for a second, unimpressed and shifting on her chair as if distracted. "Okay, I see. So, this is your version of art. Or is it something to help my mother with running her household?"

"Maybe I can answer that," came a voice from the doorway. It was Grok holding a stack of printouts. Maria thought he looked like a giant cuddly teddy bear with shaggy hair, bushy beard and a portly frame.

"You must be the famous Grok that James told me so much about," Maria said smiling, instantly warming up to the engineer.

After some hasty introductions Grok stole Maria away and initiated her into the world of computers in his cubbyhole strewn with fast food wrappers. Maria was inquisitive and curious and wasn't shy about asking questions as he put one of their new prototypes through its paces. Grok felt comfortable with her and set aside the doubts he had shared with James earlier about the wisdom of getting involved with someone whose family was against what they wanted to accomplish.

"Grok – what kind of name is that?" Maria asked teasingly.

"It's an abbreviation of my family name, Grabowski. But the word actually came from the science fiction book *Stranger in a Strange Land* where the word Grok describes the profound understanding from the deepest soulful awareness."

"Sounds intriguing."

Grok went on to explain how he met James in their early high-school days. Grok was always sharing his latest gadgets with James, who in spite of his artistic side, was also a gadget freak, always trying to make things with his engineering skills learned in school. James had even been bold enough at twelve years old to call Mr. Hewlett of Hewlett-Packard fame and ask for some spare parts for a science project. Suitably impressed, Mr. Hewlett invited James to work in a summer job at one of his factories.

A while later Grok had come across an *Esquire* magazine article about a former Air Force electronics technician named Captain Crunch who became a telecoms hacker or 'phone phreak'. Crunch figured out that the frequency from the plastic whistle in the breakfast cereal he stole his name from triggered phone company switching equipment to allow unlimited free phone calls, so he built a device to simulate the tone. Grok had to show he could do the same but using fewer microchips and built his own 'blue box'. James would assemble and sell the things at Grok's dorm in Berkeley. When Maria asked if that was against the law, Grok said they figured the phone company was already making enough money and starving students needed support. Also, Crunch used the devices to help handicapped people connect with each other so it was all pretty idealistic. Because Grok liked jokes he would do pranks like calling President Nixon claiming to be Governor Reagan, saying that there was a toilet paper shortage in California. Not reaching the president, he had just left a message with the secretary. Then he started phoning everyone from the president of France to order snails to Governor Reagan requesting him to let the Grateful Dead have a party at his mansion in Sacramento. The best was when the Pope's assistant at the Vatican put 'Henry Kissinger' on hold while he went to wake up the pontiff. Grok started to get nervous thinking the phone could be traced, so hung up before asking if the Pope was circumcised.

When Grok started to build the small computer device that was eventually Eden's main offering, he got James involved, as he was painfully shy about showing off technology, preferring to be the silent hero in the background. He intuitively knew James could market the ideas and make the general public understand their value. This lesson had been obvious with the blue boxes. The two of them as artists of the bits and bytes would go to meetings of the Homebrew Computer Club and do demos for all the other inventors.

"Like showing those funny patterns James was telling me about."

"Not only. We also got our box to play a tune by the Beatles. Anyway, these guys at the meetings were always showing off their latest inventions and sharing their tricks. There was even one guy who was proposing building a Universal Library. A global knowledge repository like one of the Seven Wonders of the World – the ancient library in Alexandria."

"How wonderful. Even my dad could understand a project like that."

"But now I'm worried we're losing our inventive spirit." The message had a meaning behind it and Maria remembered how James had explained that Grok had threatened to quit a couple of times. When the team decided to move out of the garage, Grok didn't want to go along. He thought it signaled a move from building cool machines to impress his friends to a big-time business that focused on sales and market share. James was able to talk him into coming along and quitting his full-time job but wasn't sure how long he would stay onboard.

"You sound like an artist who's forced to commercialize his work while sacrificing freedom of expression," Maria said sympathetically looking at him with caring eyes.

Grok nodded in agreement, leaning back in his office chair and linking his hands behind his head. He went on to explain his dilemma. The floodgates had opened and there was no way to get the water back now that it was flowing and nourishing a thousand new companies. The original spirit of building individual creations created camaraderie in the valley and a sense of sharing a common vision for an electronic future. Now even The Homebrew Club had changed. People wouldn't show off their designs freely unless you signed a non-disclosure agreement first, and advice that was once openly offered was held back for fear someone else will build a better device and be the first to market.

"That's really sad," Maria said wanting to give Winnie-the-Pooh a bear hug.

"Idealism is disappearing in the gold rush fever and dreams of Universal Libraries are getting lost in the race for bigger, better, faster, cheaper." He spoke with a tone of anger tinged with a hint of sadness. He reached forward to pick up a jumbo soda cup from McDonald's that was sitting in between piles of papers on his desk and took a long thoughtful pull on the straw like a child with a pacifier.

"I'm sure you and James will keep the true spirit alive. You're both so passionate about what you're doing, I know you'll find a way to preserve your vision." Grok looked at her and nodded, grateful for the reassurance.

After thanking Grok for the history lesson and technology show she found James. They left his office for a micro-vacation for the day in San Francisco, to have some time together outside their usual setting. He told his team he was meeting with suppliers and he and Maria set off for the city by the bay. Maria wanted to get to know James in a neutral environment and see if he really was a normal person who truly cared for her.

They had laughs ringing a bell on a creaking antique cable car, acting like silly tourists and then ended up in Golden Gate Park running down the hillsides pretending to be crazy kids, laughing themselves silly. At the adjacent art museum Maria explained the histories of some of the more famous paintings and James acknowledged the power of the images.

"Wow, you can really see that simplicity and form have so much power," James said in hushed tones in the large exhibit room where they stood looking at masterpieces from a variety of artists.

"Isn't it amazing how a beautiful painting transcends language? You wouldn't know the painter only spoke French," Maria said pointing to a Cézanne.

"That's right, it totally doesn't matter." James paused, quietly taking in the details and impression of the painting.

"The masters make it look so easy to create a painting that's so poetic but it took most of them a lifetime to reach that point."

"Yeah, achieving simplicity can be complicated sometimes."

After the museum tour they visited Fisherman's Wharf with the smell of the ocean and catches of fish, where the fog was burning off over the bay revealing Alcatraz Island. They slowly found their way to North Beach, a bohemian Italian neighborhood, having lunch in a small Italian restaurant Maria knew. It had red and white checkered tablecloths and Chianti bottles with candles in the neck decorating the tables. After the meal they walked arm in arm around the neighborhood window-shopping and enjoying the feeling of having no agenda, just being together making new discoveries.

"What a perfect day. This is like a dream," Maria said.

"And no pinching, I don't want to wake up from this dream. For a minute I really thought we were in Italy." As they walked along the narrow sidewalk Maria lit a cigarette and seeing James's negative look she assured him it was strictly vegetarian.

James pointed across the street. "Look, there's the Caffè Trieste where Kerouac wrote part of *On the Road*. Would be nice to sit there and write poetry for you."

"You are so sweet!"

"Come on, I'll invite you for a cappuccino." They crossed

between parked cars and he guided her to an inside table where a young lady dressed all in black took their order.

Maria pulled her chair close so she could lean her head against James's shoulder. "I'd love to take you to Italy one day. We could explore the galleries in Florence and taste real Italian cooking from my family's kitchen."

"Sounds really good. And I would like to show you India – the land of yoga and decent curries."

"On the way we could stop in Rome to meet my aunt who taught me about Tarot."

"Are you sure she wouldn't put some kind of a spell on me?"

"Don't be superstitious, she's just a wise old lady I'm very close to."

"Sounds cool – I'd like to meet her." The waitress served their coffees and they both eagerly took the cups to sample the frothy drinks.

Maria told James about some of her summers she spent with her aunt learning the old-world traditions. Running around with her cousins to *discotecas* fighting off the young Italian men (which made James briefly jealous) and swimming in the Mediterranean Sea. She inspired him with her stories of spending days in Florence soaking up the art and of the mysterious city of Venice where all the streets were canals. When he asked about her immediate family she confessed it was like the stereotype Italian dynamic. The men appearing to have all the say in things and the women quietly in the background running the household. Her parents clung to an old-world outlook from another time and place with as much dedication as they applied to their Catholic faith. Both of them hoped Maria would find a nice Italian boy to settle down with who would carry on the family tradition. The regular trips to Italy in her late teens were part of this plan. The visits actually produced the opposite effect with Maria growing into her independence and belief in her own abilities. Even though her aunt was as old-country as could be, she taught about a woman's natural power to heal and transform, which was as strong as her belief in family structure. This tradition was inspired by knowledge handed down from Roman times when women with a special connection to nature were known as witches or *venefica*, followers of Venus, the goddess associated with cultivated gardens. This meant they also used herbs for healing and love potions. The high esteem the locals in the remote mountains had for the wisdom of the goddess energy was rooted in both respect for the curative powers as well as the superstitions of the implied psychic abilities the women had from a close connection with the forces of nature. Maria never learned to ride a broomstick but chose to channel the energy she discovered through her painting as well as by developing an intuitive connection with the archetypal symbols the tarot represented.

As an only child like James, her parents revered her even though they found her ideas challenging to the way they were raised. Her parents accepted that being in the last reaches of Western civilizations meant some adaptation to evolution was necessary. They still held out hope for her to marry a young man of similar background. While Tobias may not have been an ideal candidate, he had some of the characteristics of the type of partner they imagined. This theme was still a perennial issue that was discussed over the family dinners on Sunday much to Maria's dislike. All in all, her relationship with her parents was harmonious but existed on the basis of an uneasy truce. As she was in her early twenties they accepted that at her age she would have more independence and that their ability to influence was limited.

"What about your family? You know all about mine for better or for worse. My father is not as bad as you imagine. He really does have a big heart." Maria took a sip from her coffee and looked at James over the top of her cup.

James smiled and said he was sure her father was a good man to have raised such a fine daughter which earned him a playful punch on the arm. He described briefly his childhood that he characterized as a typical suburban upbringing with caring parents who supported his every interest. His stepfather was always working on fixing up cars, so James learned a lot of his skills in building things and negotiating for parts from watching his father operate. He gave a brief recap of his college time in a liberal arts college where he learned calligraphy and got deep into Eastern religion that led to his trip to India he had explained to her in earlier conversations.

The conversation had reached a comfortable pause and Maria paid for the coffees, being a liberated lady. "I know a great gelato place around the corner. Ready for dessert?" Maria asked, happy to be together.

James shifted uncomfortably in his seat averting his eyes, afraid to break the feeling of closeness that had developed. "I would love to. This day is so magical," he said unconvincingly.

"But…" Maria said with a tone of anger mixed with disappointment knowing what was coming and looking at him seriously to hear what bomb he was going to drop this time.

James let out a sigh and started his explanation in a defeated tone. "I need to slowly head back to the office." Maria had a watchful look and leaned back crossing her arms over her chest. "The board are expecting big profits this quarter to justify more funding. I'm already playing hooky to be here." He said it reluctantly knowing Maria had made a similar sacrifice and had lied to her parents about where she was. James had subconsciously shifted his attention back to his primary focus like flipping a switch on a circuit. If Eden Computers was his attempt at creating a more perfect world then was Maria offering the apple of temptation that would distract him from his dream and cast him among the mortals? At the same time this thought flashed through James's mind Maria was wondering if their two very different worlds and backgrounds could find a livable middle ground. A part of her accepted James's quirkiness when it came to technology as another aspect of his artistic nature but it was the eyes of a farmer's daughter that were watching.

James looked at her studying him with pleading eyes and his resistance melted. He smiled and leaned over, kissing her quickly on the cheek. "You're really too much. How am I supposed to get anything done when I'm powerless to say no?" They both laughed. "I think I'm a victim of one of those magic spells your aunt taught you."

"You catch on quickly for a city boy," Maria said smiling slyly.

"How about we meet in the middle – we go for gelato and then head home? I would love for this afternoon to go on forever but I can't ignore the business too long."

"I agree on one condition. Next time we go to the opera and stay overnight."

James took her hand. "You really are a good negotiator. I think you should be working for me."

11

BLEM GARDENS

Stephan liked to think that while 1920s Hollywood had its Garden of Allah, 1970s West LA had its Blem Gardens. While the Allah hosted the likes of Bogie and Bacall, Garbo and Dietrich, Fitzgerald and Hemingway and all of the Marx Brothers, Blem was home to its own creative circle, talented but unknown. Okay, there was no swimming pool with a naked Marilyn floating in it, but it had other quaint characters to compensate. A couple of paint-splattered artists, a scrambling screenwriter and half of a rock and roll band all waiting for their friend fame to find them.

Located one block away from the border of Santa Monica, on a small residential street of old houses and eight- or ten-unit apartment buildings from the fifties, Blem Gardens was in a time warp, close in age and size to its more famous Hollywood cousin. The Gardens was a courtyard of six bungalows, three on each side of a broad drive that ended in a weed-choked yard. For his loyalty as an early supporter of Jiva, Stephan had graciously been invited by the band's manager to take over a bungalow after the band had scattered from the Echo Park house to live their individual lives. The name for the cluster of former vacation cabanas originated from Jiva's lead guitarist, who saw the combination of funky architecture and enlightened natives as a creative melting pot.

Jim, an artist from Philadelphia, occupied the bungalow closest to the street on the south side of the gardens. He had converted his living room into one large studio with paintings hanging on every wall in various stages of completion and stacked five or six deep in other places. Worktables completed the décor, covered with baby food jars, each holding a custom-created color. Jim worked day and night with a stereo blasting music while he created large acrylic compositions of geometric shapes and strange angles inspired by Richard Diebenkorn, another migrant painter based downtown. Jim kept his hair conservatively short and customarily wore paint-covered white overalls. He would randomly choose a neighbor to share a joint with when his inspiration faded. He had recently taken up surfing and was proud of his night trips to Malibu to surf in the dark at County Line with punk musicians, adding to a visible attitude he wanted to cultivate as part of his persona.

Across from Jim there was another artist in residence with her husband. Melony and John were newlyweds in their twenties. While he was a frumpy grade school teacher usually attired in Pendleton plaid and work boots, Melony was a fringe fan of the burgeoning punk music scene that she had grown close to while studying art at West LA College. She dressed and acted accordingly. Miniskirts, tall boots and lots of black were her trademark that complemented her trim, petite frame and pretty face. Her paintings and sketches were not as bold as Jim's but had a defined character that the portraits personified in brooding compositions.

The bungalow in-between Melony and Stephan was home to a screenwriter named Maceo who would act like a hermit and not appear for days when he was deep into polishing a draft of a new project. The neighbors only saw him when he came and went from his day job as a reservation's operator for British Airways at their call center by Westwood. Maceo focused on retelling American history from an idealistic perspective. He and the band members often drank beer on his breaks from creativity and had political debates on the state of the country and how it got to be such an appalling mess.

Next to Jim's bungalow Jiva's lead singer Michael lived with his gorgeous blond wife. When not writing songs, he was on the front porch holding court on whatever latest political scandal was unveiling. His wife Adrienne worked as a receptionist at a doctor's office with a predictable routine that balanced out Michael's more erratic schedule of late nights and equally late mornings. The last bungalow in the row that faced Stephan's new home was where Jack the band manager and Reedo the drummer lived in bachelor splendor. Visitors were greeted in the living room by one of the twelve million Farrah Fawcett red swimsuit posters that heralded her role on the opening season of *Charlie's Angels*.

On a Sunday afternoon, warmed by diffused sunlight that made the whole world seem lazy, Stephan escaped the smell of carbonized toast he had burned for breakfast. He wandered over to Maceo's bungalow to talk shop and compare notes on their writing projects. Mac had never sold a film script but was sure he was onto the next big thing – the ultimate bicentennial story of an astronaut hero running for president who gets caught up in a fight with a large corporation trying to take over Native American land. He hoped to finish it in time to make a killing as a tie-in to the patriotic mood built up by this year's 1776 two-hundred-year birthday celebrations of the country. Stephan had been acting informally as a script consultant, giving pointers on the story structure and character development.

Stephan climbed the sagging stairs to the weather-beaten porch and stuck his head in the dim living room, as the front door was open. He saw Mac writing out some notes from a book about the great pyramid. A few years older than Stephan, he looked like a junior professor, with a prematurely receding hairline and polo shirt that went with his no-nonsense attitude.

"Hey, man, is it safe to come in?" Stephan asked.

"Who are you, an Amway salesman or a Jehovah's Witness?"

"Sorry, just a fellow scribe in search of motivation."

"I hate to be the bearer of bad tidings, but the pot's all gone and I'm drinking the last beer."

Stephan moved an empty pizza box off the small sofa jammed against the wall and sat down. "Damn, I'll have to get by with caffeine then. Got any coffee?"

Mac tore a corner from his notebook page to mark the place in the pyramid book he was studying. He went to get some coffee from the Mr. Coffee machine that was always switched on with a pot of evil-smelling brew perpetually warming up.

He called out from the kitchen, "Did you know that on the dollar bill, the pyramid on the Great Seal has thirteen levels? The eagle on the other half has thirteen tail feathers, the olive branch has thirteen olives and there are a lot of other thirteens. If you ask me, the Masonic influences are obvious. The Founding Fathers were not just politicians but mystic visionaries."

"I hope you can get that message across, because after Nixon in the White House anyone else will be a saint. The new guy Carter is a start. Someone who can command a submarine and invite the Allman Brothers to Washington for the inauguration can't be all bad. We need to make peace with Russia before World War Three kicks off." Stephan directed his words in the direction of the kitchen that due to the small size of the house was next to where he was sitting and meant he didn't have to raise his voice. He picked up a well-worn book on the American Revolution sitting next to him and thumbed through it.

"Did I tell you what our lovely neighbor Lady Melony was doing last week?" Maceo said coming back into the living room. He handing Stephan a mug of coffee decorated with a peace sign filled in with stars and stripes.

"No, do tell. I'm overdue for a visit."

"Dream on, don't forget she's married," Maceo said sitting down at his desk.

"Yeah, but I think she likes me."

"Join the club. Anyway, I'm on my way back from the

market one afternoon and I notice her door is open. I walk over to where I can look in and say howdy and what do I see? Melony sitting on the living room floor sketching her vagina with the help of a mirror."

"You're joking."

"Swear to God. Looked like an exotic orchid. I say 'hi' and she looks up and says she's doing her homework for an anatomy class."

"She invite you in?"

"Come on, she's a respectable woman." They both laughed. "Hey, I don't want to be a rude host but I got to see my folks for Sunday dinner." Maceo shuffled some papers together to make a neat stack.

"Bon appetite, amigo," Stephan said knocking back the remains of the tepid coffee in one swallow.

Stephan started back to his bungalow and saw Reedo framed in the doorway of the opposite small house tapping his drumsticks on a practice pad while watching TV. Reedo nodded a greeting and Stephan was happy to continue procrastinating and wandered over.

"What's going on, man?" Reedo asked with his eyes locked on a rerun of $M*A*S*H$ with its sporadic laugh track, while he tapped a nervous staccato beat.

"Same old, same old. Trying to bring home the wisdom of the East." Stephan leaned back on the ancient wood front porch railing and stuck his hands in his jeans pockets.

"Hear anything from Greasy since he split?"

"Nothing, but then he's not the letter-writing type. I'll chase him down in a few weeks when I go see my folks. When's your next gig?"

"Wednesday, at the Corral up in Topanga. Don't miss it. I invited some cuties from the skate club in Hollywood." Reedo looked over at Stephan with a smile as he continued his drumming.

"What's that, the roller derby?"

Reedo stopped his practicing and held the drumsticks still against the practice pad as he relived his memories describing the scene. "Nothing like you've ever seen. It's a remodeled roller-skating rink called the Starlight where you skate around to disco music and there are some awesome babes, I can tell you. Last week Cher was boogying around. I met some chicks there that want to hear us play, so be sure to iron your undies if you want to score. One of them is an awesome British chick who's been to some of our gigs already. The bummer is she's married." Reedo shook his head in disappointment.

"But she has friends," Stephan said getting a knowing grin in return.

"Oh yeah. Some real naughty nookie," Reedo answered with a mischievous smile.

"I'll be there. I want to hear you play 'Kabir's Blues' again. Where's Jack? I see the Toad is gone." Stephan was referring to a monster twin cab pickup truck that was usually parked behind the bungalow on the small lawn. The off-road vehicle looked like it had been abandoned by the military with the color of a desert frog.

"He's doing his desert-rat thing out in the Mojave with a buddy. If they're not looking for gold, they're getting drunk and shooting at the empties."

Reedo was an Air Force brat and his energetic rock and

roll persona was tamed by a quality of inner discipline he sought to shape from a military seriousness to a creative focus. His small frame was topped by a shoulder-length set of big hair popular with the more successful bands like Van Halen who were playing around town. He loved to play music but groupies came a close second in his list of favorite things. He was continually looking at new ways to meet female music fans and worked out in a gym so his physique could aid him in his quest.

Jack had also shared an Air Force background, as San Bernardino hosted a couple of squadrons of pilots. He had been the band's mentor and father figure in its early stages gigging around the area, and after winning some local Battle of the Band contests he talked them into finding fame and fortune in the music capital of the universe, an hour's drive to the north. It was an easy escape from a dusty, windblown and smoggy town where opportunities as a musician were seriously limited.

To pay the bills, Jack worked on special effects for director Roger Corman's B-movie science fiction flicks, turning toaster ovens into spaceports and stereo components into death rays; Jack was a wizard with electronics gear. The TV was perpetually on in their bungalow and the kitchen was a shrine to undying bachelorhood. The centerpiece was a frying pan coated with remnants of the previous day's dinner grease. Jack maintained a collection of the most amazing porno magazines that anyone had ever seen, sharing them on rare occasions with select neighbors. He had a kindness and patience that came from being ten years more senior than the oldest band member and this more mature attitude helped secure gigs that a young, longhaired musician couldn't.

Jack had originally discovered Jiva when he had done the wiring and electronics installation for a friend's recording studio and needed to hire some real, live musicians to test the set-up. His roommate's sister was dating the lead guitarist, so an arrangement was made for the band to get a free demo tape in exchange for being the guinea pigs to help iron out the kinks in the studio's acoustics. It was every band's dream and they quickly accepted the offer.

Jack was extremely impressed by their musicianship and offered to manage them. He liked their sound because it was clean, strong and original, with no standards or tunes from the Top Forty. Under Jack's management they went on to win several contests, with the usual prize an amplifier or speakers, but they were rapidly outgrowing their territory.

Moving north, they did the usual round of LA club gigs, rocking the public with highly danceable tunes. They managed to get into the Whisky A Go Go, hoping to be the latest hot discovery like The Doors, who had been the house band for a while until their song 'Light My Fire' made it to number one on the singles charts. Michael, the lead singer had the spirit and passion of English soul singer Joe Cocker complete with spastic animation and would easily get lost in belting out a song. His emotional range covered everything from a tear-jerking ballad to a humorous sing-along.

Reedo was the driving force behind the band and put out a consistent beat to push the music along, with a tight syncopation that was at times a frenzy of flailing drumsticks while other times a smooth rhythm. Tommy, their slinky guitarist, with trendy haircut including bangs and fluffed-up top had lightning-fast fingers. He traded licks with a tall, serious-looking bass player named Jim, who thumped out a rhythmic groove in synch with Reedo and rounded out the band.

When the band first moved to LA as teenagers just out of high school, they all shared a big Victorian house in Echo Park off of Sunset where it made its large turn towards downtown through run-down stores. It was a corner of the city that time forgot and had let slide into obscurity. The shopfronts looked like they hadn't changed since the 1950s, and the houses had remained in a time warp giving a view of what LA was like during a time of optimistic prosperity and ambitious plans of classic architecture and sophisticated styling for that time. Nothing more had happened since then, so the homes gave the impression they were leaning on each other to keep from falling down. Jack paid a lion's share of the rent as he was the most qualified to find a paying gig. The nights were always a party scene, with the band members and their groupies who evolved into girlfriends providing enough of a catalyst to attract anyone looking to have some fun in a rambling old house with huge garden. The band was living there when Stephan and Greasy met them at a show by the beach, and afterwards the two of them were quickly integrated into the extended family as roadies and mechanic. Having moved on from Echo Park into a more mature phase of individual households, the band now rehearsed most nights in a garage not far from the old house.

The band adopted their name after their move to LA when the band members started to practice meditation after meeting a teacher from India. The name was a Hindi word meaning 'that which breathes', commonly used to signify the individual soul; the drop of the ocean that has the same qualities of the infinite ocean. Jiva built up a core group of dedicated fans that went wild at all their shows, dancing from the first song all the way through a series of encores. Willing teenage girls from the Valley ended up as groupies, with each band member eventually getting lucky with a foxy blond or some Valley Girl with killer curves who used 'totally' and 'whatever' in every sentence. And yet the ever-elusive record contract was nowhere to be found, so they kept at it, working their odd jobs until a deal would finally come through. Even with the help of musicians they knew playing around town, or friends like the soundman at the Troubadour, and the doorman at the Roxy it didn't help, as the competition to get a deal was fierce.

As good fortune sometimes smiles on those who persevere and have talent, someone eventually recognized them. The first person with some influence to take them seriously was a British fan named Trish, who danced herself silly at their shows as an antidote to her stuffy ruling-class upbringing and accompanying hereditary title. Trish had been slumming in the Whisky one night and was so enamored with Jiva's music that she and her girlfriends danced like pagan celebrants. They kept Reedo smiling and slightly distracted and were a boon for Stephan and the other guys on the dance floor.

The band had launched into their trademark song

'Take My Love' with a slowly building guitar riff of R & B flavored funk, joined by the thump of the bass that was reminiscent of the galloping drive of reggae, and nobody could sit still. By the time Michael started belting out the first lines, the dance floor was packed.

Open the door that turns the key to your heart
You're something special, you've a load to uncart
What do you know about lying
What do you know about dying
What do you say we start trying
To unwind
The sign of the times
It's not hard
It starts in your own yard
Take my love
Wear it well
Take my love
It's too soon tell
How far we can go
With love

Michael started scat singing over a guitar solo that merged into a bass line that the drums picked up and pushed onward, and then the whole band blasted into the next verse. The club's wooden floor was pulsating like a giant drum skin and bottles and glasses were rattling on tables. The public matched the increasing insistency of the beat driven by a thundering bass and clanging guitar with frantic tribal dance rhythms. By the time the next verse had gone by and the chorus started, the whole club was shouting 'take my love', clapping and stomping along.

Stephan had a small share in the band's fortunes, having given them a couple of short poems to use as songs. One was called Kabir's Blues, based on the 16th century mystic's poetry. The other was about a blind date Malone had recently organized for him that ended with disastrous results and he had called the piece 'One Out of Three'. It referred to how the mystery lady described herself – tall, blond and attractive. In the end she was only blond, and even that wasn't her natural color.

Michael liked both poems and set them to music and they became part of their repertoire. Michael was always encouraging Stephan's writing and said that the rhymes were good signs of his creative potential. And besides, with a number one hit, a songwriter could live off the residuals for a long time. Michael hadn't been impressed with Malone's astrological rap or shady schemes and was always encouraging Stephan to have courage and jump into his writing with both feet. At the same time, he sympathized with trying to do this while needing a day job.

At one of the band's next gigs Trish brought along her former husband, Alan, whose main claim to fame was organizing the Monterey Pop Festival. He had also managed a variety of British musicians in the early sixties and was well known as a bad boy around town for partying away his inheritance while racing around town in his Dino Ferrari. He checked Jiva out and was impressed enough to sign on to represent them. He got the band's first self-recorded LP in front of one of his British mates, George Harrison, who was interested enough to go to one of their shows with his dark, sweet Latina lady who had already heard the band play. George spoke to the band afterwards and said the energy reminded him of his early days with the Beatles. A few days after the concert, Harrison set up a formal meeting to meet the band at the offices of his record label, Dark Horse Records. It was located in one of the small buildings on the A&M Records lot, the parent company handling marketing and distribution. They all had a few laughs getting to know each other and George predicted Jiva would do all right. He suggested borrowing a friend of his who was a successful keyboardist with a hot single called *Dreamweaver* to provide some backup. Jack and Alan acting as co-managers handled the negotiations and, in a few weeks, they were offered a contract.

Later, Jack had a meeting with George to iron out some details of joining his record label, and George in his low-key style mentioned to Jack that he hoped Alan wouldn't fumble this one. Not catching the full portent of this comment, the negotiations continued and a final deal was agreed with Jiva becoming the first American band signed to Dark Horse Records. An energetic and efficient young lady named Hart Akers was assigned to support the band and within a week Jiva went off to the Record Plant to make their first album.

12

IT'S ONLY A NORTHERN SONG

Stephan flew north to visit his parents for his father's birthday with the idea of checking on Greg and James. After the obligatory family dinner with his parents and sisters, Stephan borrowed his dad's Pinto and started to make the rounds, beginning with James. It was easy to locate him because his focus on the company meant he could always be found in the Eden offices day and night. When Stephan arrived, James was presiding over a meeting of his engineers, so Stephan found his way to the bare-bones waiting room reading some out-of-date electronics magazines. A short while later he saw the engineers returning to their cubicles and went searching for James. Stephan nodded to a few engineers he had worked with at Atari the previous summer to get his India money together. Everyone was too concentrated on their assembly or development work to talk, and Stephan ended up waiting for James to get off the phone. He wasn't surprised to hear him forcefully directing orders at a supplier who was late delivering components.

"So please remind me again what I got to do to get my parts. You want the first twenty machines off the assembly line for you and your pals or do I go to my contacts in

Japan?" After hearing a response, he said a quick thanks and tossed the phone into the cradle. Looking at Stephan standing in the door he caught his breath and said, "Well, hi there. The wandering monk returns. You finish your book?"

Stephan took a seat on a folding chair by the desk and explained that the Rama epic was still a work in progress but he'd adapted some of his poetry as songs for some neighbors who were in a band. "If I'm lucky they might even put it on an album they're recording. Can you believe it – they were signed by one of the Beatles!"

"Very cool," James said respectfully as he searched through a stack of papers.

Stephan carried on. "And speaking of books, I'm working with somebody who is going to reveal to the world all the secrets of tantric massage."

James stopped his rummaging and looked at Stephan with admiration for hitting on something sensible sounding. "Now you're talking. Forget that spiritual mumbo jumbo, give the people what they want. And right now, sex sells."

James offered Stephan a rice cake that looked like molded Styrofoam and explained he had started a macrobiotic diet to balance his energies. Stephan asked if the raw-foods diet was history as it was James's earlier belief that uncooked foods were closer to the natural order of humans' original diet. But James had said the Japanese had perfected a better system. Grok had been listening from the doorway waiting to give James a report.

"Yeah, and bathing washes away all our natural oils, leaving us open to disease," he said imitating James. "Don't knock it, Stephan, at least he washes now and is laying off the raw garlic body scrubs. I'm guessing it has more to do with his lady than his health." He tossed the papers on James's desk and left with James giving the finger to Grok's disappearing back. Grok looked back and caught Stephan's eye and nodded in the direction of his work area on the shop floor, indicating an invite to stop by.

"From the look of things business is booming. Maybe I should buy one of these computers for my company. Can I get a discount?" Stephan asked.

"I'm not running a charity here. If I give everyone I know a break I'll go broke," James said with a grin.

"No worries – my business is also taking off, so I can put one in the budget."

"Let me give you a demo." James started up a machine on a small typing table while Stephan stood next to him and watched various messages appear on the screen.

"Why is it telling us to wait? I thought we were supposed to tell it what to do, but the machine looks like it's the boss," Stephan said.

"That's just the operating system loading. We're fixing that so the machine will be ready in under five minutes." James turned away from the machine and grabbed the bag of rice cakes off his desk.

"Sounds cool. How's your lady?" Stephan asked looking around the cluttered office and spying a painting on one wall.

"Beautiful as ever. She's busier than I am if you can believe it. There's one of her latest creations." James pointed to the vibrant watercolor of some fall trees changing their foliage, hanging between some schematic diagrams taped on the wall that Stephan had been observing.

Stephan stepped closer to the picture, admiring it. "Nice."

"Okay, here we go." The demo machine had finally got to a blinking cursor on a blank screen, so James clacked on the keyboard entering some commands. A new string of text appeared and started scrolling from top to bottom and James cursed. "Demo effect. Just when you want it to work, it's looping."

"No problem, I'll check it out next time. What's it supposed to do?"

James turned to Stephan and was making gestures like a professor in a lecture hall. "We've got this program based on an idea we stole from the Xerox research lab. The concept is that what you type appears on the screen and the cool part is you can mark the words and move them from one place to another or change the font and some other neat stuff."

"Nice. Could use that for sure in my publishing work. And then? How do I get it onto paper?"

"You need a printing device."

"Okay…"

"Look, I can't go into it right now without you signing an NDA, but we're also working on another technology from the same lab. It's under wraps right now, so I can't even give you a clue. But trust me it's big. We're going to blow the minds of the business world. The management back east thought the Xerox lab was a bunch of stoned California hippies making fun toys and completely missed what all their millions in development money were producing."

"One of your engineers told me they really were a bunch

of freaks who sat in a circle smoking dope and drinking wine to brainstorm."

"Like, who cares? Don't judge a book by its cover." They both laughed. "Those guys made an operating system that's so easy to use, with little pictures to represent the things you can do. They also made it possible to send the text you type to another person on the other side of the planet."

"They really did that?" Stephan said with awe, his eyes wide in mock disbelief.

"Very cool shit. But listen; more importantly we're going to revolutionize education. These new machines will be easy enough for a kid to use and will make learning so much fun. And at the same time, we'll be making the kids smarter than their parents ever were. We're speeding up human evolution." James was standing now as he excitedly expressed his vision.

"Whoa – that little box can do all that? But what about personal development?"

"I know what you're getting at. You're gonna tell me the baba said we should work on our inner focus. I haven't forgotten. I work on my personal satori or enlightenment whenever I can. I've got a little routine going on down at the Zen center. How about you?" James moved back to his desk and was looking at his agenda.

"Still researching Indian texts to get some ideas for my story. Catching a few yoga classes and some meditation here and there. Now I'm heading over the hill to see Greg. You seen him lately?"

"All I hear is occasional second-hand news from our mechanic buddy Frank. When Greg first moved back, I saw him on and off when he would stop by for a coffee, but it was always a bit awkward. Neither one of us was sure if we could apologize enough to move on from the race story. It's sad because the three of us were real tight." James had shifted his sales pitch voice to a softer, more thoughtful tone. "Remember all those all-night rap sessions trying to figure out the meaning of the universe? He used to be like our local teacher and now he's got some hustle going on with Bernie I don't want to know about."

"Doesn't sound like a way to keep out of trouble."

"I'm trying to help by letting him do yoga classes in my new house in Los Gatos. Maria brings some of her friends along, so he's king of the hill again with a room full of young ladies hanging on his every word."

"And what about the risk from Tobias's father wanting payback?" Stephan asked.

"Nothing's happened until now and it's been close to six months. I haven't heard anything, and to be honest, I haven't been thinking about it. I've got enough on my plate with this outfit to worry about." He pulled his phone closer. "Sorry to be in a rush, but time is money and I've got customers waiting. Why don't you stop by my place tomorrow for dinner? Can check out the new hacienda and say hi to Maria."

"That'd be cool but I need to get back to LA tomorrow. Another time."

"No problem. See you around then." He smiled and reached over to where Stephan was sitting and they quickly did the soul shake. Then he swung around on his chair, reached for his phone and quickly dialed a number, cranking the rotor with a pencil. Stephan felt like another vendor on a courtesy call whose presence wasn't required any more.

Stephan got up, headed for the door and said, "Namaste, brother," folding his hands in front of his heart, getting the flash of a peace sign from James in return.

Stephan looked around and found Grok's cubicle where he assembled prototypes in the back of the workroom. He leaned over, resting his elbows on the low wall for a quick chat. Grok was fiddling with a circuit board, inspecting it from all angles. The air smelled of burnt solder from the soldering iron heating in its stand and that clinical metallic smell of electronic circuits.

"Things sure have come a long way since I last saw your operation," Stephan said as he looked up across the large workroom.

"I think you saw the best of times when it wasn't about market share or keeping the investors happy." Grok deftly pulled a transistor from the board with some needle-nose pliers.

"It's a hard balance to find between inspiration and paying the rent."

"I could go back to Hewlett-Packard and do my fun stuff in my spare time just as easy," Grok said with his face obscured by the board he was scrutinizing.

"Maybe, but it would always be someone else's ideas you're developing. And now with all the electronic companies taking off, you have a chance to shape the industry like you want."

Grok leaned back in his chair looking at Stephan. "It feels like we've lost our innocence and replaced it with a desire for material gain." He reached for a large white Slurpee cup with the 7-Eleven logo on it and took a long drink, replacing the cup carefully on a teetering stack of printouts.

"Then remember those ideals you were all talking about. You're really an enabler of change for the masses which is not at all an insignificant effort."

"Tell James – he's the one who seems the most lost in all the push by our new investors to show results." Grok shook his head in defeat.

"I'll work on it but you shouldn't forget your focus. After all you are the one with the crazy ideas that translate into what people want with James's creative flair."

"Thanks, man – I'll keep looking towards the blue sky." He smiled affirmatively at Stephan and turned to hunch over the problem circuit board.

Stephan pushed away from the low wall with a friendly "see ya later" and found his way out.

A couple of months earlier on his return north Greg had made a very low-key landing at a commune of yogis. It was located on Trout Gulch Road, somewhere between Santa Cruz and Los Gatos, where the coastal foothills rolled towards the looming mountain range.

To further keep off the local radar Greasy had adopted a new handle, calling himself Shri Das, and wore a dhoti accented by a wizened beatnik beard and crew-cut hair. The beard and short hair were an intentional disguise as Greg didn't want to take any chances being in the same vicinity of the people who wanted him crucified. Shri Das gave the karma dharma farmer rap to any of his friends like Bernie who were patient enough to listen from over a glass of freshly squeezed beet juice. The talk was Greg's usual mile-a-minute monologue, with the mix of humor, mysticism and social commentary. Greg and his fellow yogis were hardcore vegetarians and their house was a collection of sleeping bags on the bedroom floors in an otherwise orderly middle-class home, with the followers doing a variety of day jobs to pay the rent. The yogi monk phase of Greg's life had ended after a month when he felt it was safe to circulate once again while keeping out of sight. Ever since moving back up north, Greg slowly convinced himself that the DiFilippo's anger had cooled and that they believed he had left the state. With a confident attitude he started to freely move on the periphery of society, in the Valley and over at the beach.

When Stephan tracked down Greg, he found him living in an apartment in the anonymous lower middle-class suburbs of Santa Cruz by the yacht harbor, with a cute girlfriend who worked as a nurse somewhere. Greg had decided to avoid a mechanic's job to not be too obvious and now dabbled in haircutting, thinking it may be a new career opportunity. The reigning style was long hair in the back, almost to the shoulder, short sides and thick top with a kind of bangs in the front. It was a unisex style of Glam Rock, big heels and sparkling, skintight clothes that a freaked-out spaceman would wear. The less glamorous name for it was 'the mullet'. Greg wouldn't let Stephan get by without a styling, which made Stephan part of the gang, and would no doubt set his usual LA hair stylist's teeth on edge.

While Greg moved around the chair working on Stephan's hair, he rapped in a knowledgeable tone about how he was slowly getting back to normal and how he was working on rebuilding some old cars in his garage.

"Good to hear. You get any sense of people around here gunning for you?" Stephan asked trying to keep his head straight so a part of his ear didn't get snipped off.

"I've been all over this town and nobody's given me the time of day. The only person who knows what I look like is Tobias's dad and friends, and all the friends are mostly from San Francisco where he went to school, so no worries. Anyway, I spend most of my time over in the Valley where I'm just one more ugly mug cruising in an old Chevy."

Stephan warned, "All the same take it easy, 'cause the dad will go crazy if he hears you're around."

"Even Maria ain't heard a word, so it looks like the storm has blown over. I see that gal every week when I teach her and her little Saratoga honeys a few asanas."

"Yeah, but knowing that she's friends with some of us, would her family really tell her anything?" Stephan wisely pointed out.

"I think she'd hear something," Greg assured him. "I can see why James hooked up with her – the sweetest goddess around. Gives me the female view of the universe and some damn good advice to boot."

"Yeah, I'm going to miss not seeing her this trip. She's a very cool lady."

Stephan made the rounds with Greg, including Santa

Cruz's best-known disco, the Dragon Moon, where Greg had established himself as a name there in one of his disguises as a disco prince. He would wear stylish clothes and contact lenses, a far cry from his former look of a denim-shirt-clad auto mechanic with working-class-hero glasses. That look was a thing of the past. He was frequently getting warned and temporarily banned for dancing too dirty with his girlfriend in a repeat of his show at the DiFilippo club.

Another platform for Greg to show off was at showings of *The Rocky Horror Picture Show*. It was a regular midnight movie that he and his girlfriend knew all the songs to and would pantomime the scenes in the aisles. Greg would dress as Riff Raff, the scraggly butler and his girlfriend like Magenta, complete with French maid costume and hot pants. They would dance and sing snippets of songs with the groups of revelers waiting to get in. It was as much a show as the movie itself with Greg as the main cheerleader, working the crowd up for the event.

There was nothing associated with sex Greg didn't know or hadn't done, so a blatant exhibition of his free attitude on the dance floor was expected. Greg freely admitted he had experimented with threesomes and foursomes leading to a gay encounter with a hairdresser who hung around the fringe of Greasy's circle of friends. Stephan guessed the gay experience was a short-term experiment; Greg explored any and all possibilities, pushing the boundaries wherever he could.

In Santa Cruz, the police were busy trying to handle a nonstop stream of transients who had heard that the spirit of the sixties lived on in the small coastal town. The rugged landscape and tradition of independence allowed for many small pockets of criminality, from small-time pot farmers in the mountains harvesting their cash crops to fishing boats that picked up hundreds of pounds of Mexican grass or cocaine from trawlers venturing into the main Pacific shipping lanes. Invariably, some of the smaller change doing little hustles like Greg fell through the cracks. Greasy was able to surf this channel and move and groove to whatever rhythms were going on. Everybody seemed to be his friend and with enough connections around town, he was always running one deal or another. Sometimes it was car parts, other times it was some herbal remedies of both the legal and contraband version.

Lunch the next day was nachos and beer at the Tampico Kitchen on the less sophisticated end of the tree-lined pedestrian mall that ran through the downtown area. Following that came a trip to the Catalyst, a Wild West bar full of old hippies and freshly scrubbed university kids who bumped around to local bands. Tonight's concert would feature a group called The Ducks with the local native Neil Young jamming along. The phenomenal amount of beer consumed soon put a glaze on Stephan's eyes. Greg was finally so loaded he simply slid down the stairs from the balcony in one fluid movement, not attracting the slightest attention – he was always doing something unusual.

Stephan knew it was the moment to leave when a waiter looking like the biggest freak in the place told him to put out a joint. Stephan had tried to hand it to the waiter thinking he was looking for a puff. The other people at the table who had shared it with him thought he was totally uncool and lectured him about his indiscretion.

The next morning Stephan and Greg were admiring a collection of car parts in the backyard, sitting on some sagging plastic lawn chairs while recovering with a pot of coffee. The hangover was humbling and Greg let down his front a little.

"You know, after my LA experience I saw working on cars wasn't the most desirable pastime. I've slowed down on twisting wrenches and busting bolts to pay the rent. For fun, I still like to rebuild motors to increase their performance and then make test runs on the Coast Highway."

Stephan knew from an earlier talk with their mechanic buddy Frank that he usually ended up doing the bulk of the work at his compound in the foothills above Cupertino. Greg's attention span couldn't keep him focused long enough to see a project through to completion. Frank always was the better mechanic anyway, with more tools and experience, while Greg preferred the racing and comparing of autos with other mechanics. They still talked about opening a garage and calling it Karmic Annex, but like a flea on a hot frying pan, Greg could never sit still long enough to iron out the details.

Greg had managed to wheel and deal and put together a fleet of old Dodge Darts, Plymouth Valiants and Chevy pickups. He was pulling in some phenomenal amounts of money driving for Bernie, who was now based in Marin, dealing in various illegal substances, mostly 'speed' or 'crank'. Bernie had been active over the years in a variety of schemes both legal and illegal. He was always looking for the least amount of work for the most reward, with his latest efforts tending towards the latter. Worm farms and India imports didn't have the same high return as illegal substances. Greg explained that speed was as innocent as the diet pills doctors prescribed, always the drug of choice for blue-collar workers and truck drivers. When he was in mechanics school, the bikers and other greaseballs always had some. Even housewives were using it to lose weight and getting so wired you'd think they were plugged into an electric outlet the way they cleaned their houses at an accelerated rate.

Stephan added that the first time he was offered crank was at an Atari party where some of the engineers needed the extra boost to pull all-nighters. Stephan had the urge to add something about the perils of getting into the drug scene, but was reluctant to sound like a preacher as he had earlier that day. The world Greg moved in meant there were more funny white powders being offered, and Greg's disappearing periodically for private meetings with friends maybe wasn't just to talk business. But in the end, Stephan kept quiet.

"Bernie's moved on from Los Gatos to this palatial home on the side of Mount Tamalpais totally hidden somewhere above San Anselmo. Got a mind-blowing view of San Francisco."

"It's definitely where I'd go if I had the cash. Guess he needs the privacy so the neighbors don't get too curious."

Greg explained that Bernie had done a year of jail time for a grass deal gone bad back in 1970. He wanted to avoid any further incidents that would land him in a penitentiary rather than the low security jail he was in for his first offence. He said that he felt the dynamic had shifted with Bernie now playing the boss, considering Greg more of an employee than a friend. The risk was all on Greg, but the money was mostly Bernie's. Greg loved to rile him by tuning in a classic station on his B&O stereo with hidden speakers and always got a laugh seeing Bernie swearing, tripping all over his Afghani caftan on the way to the stereo controls asking who turned on the fag music.

In the six months he had been away a lot had changed and Greg regretted the awkwardness of reconnecting with James. It was like they were getting to know each other again for the first time only with the handicap of a shared tragedy coloring their efforts. Maria had been helpful trying to bridge the differences, and if anything, Greg had gotten to know her better in the past months than James. Greg felt he had moved on from the accident. If anybody was still stuck on the incident it was James who tried to ignore dealing with it by working day and night. Greg suspected one of the reasons James couldn't let it go was he was reminded of the race every time he saw Maria. Even though the two were growing closer, the possibility to make total peace with her and to win her family's acceptance was blocked because of Tobias's death.

Greg changed the subject. "Sounds like LA is treating you mighty fine. I sure hope things also turn around for me 'cause right now I'm holding back so the wrong people don't notice."

"Give it some more time. The race will eventually be part of history. Those guys have other stuff to worry about."

"Sure hope so. Now remember what I said about that

Malone guy – don't place all your bets on just one horse. And whenever you get bored down south let me know – we still have that yoga center to set-up. Got a little property up north I have my eye on."

The reunion ended on a quiet note, as Stephan had to get back over to the valley for his flight home. The monstrous hangovers made them part like war-weary soldiers off to start another campaign. Stephan had hoped to return to LA reassured Greg was doing well but the feeling was more of a ticking time bomb with an inevitable explosion somewhere down the road. He knew Greg was not the type to stay quiet for too long and the more driving he did for Bernie, the more opportunities there were to be noticed. And even though Maria and her friends could be trusted to keep quiet about the yoga classes, the valley had eyes and ears. As the Pinto shimmied around the curves heading through the deeply forested mountains Stephan felt resigned to letting the universe unfold in whatever way was destined for him and his friends. He was hoping that the compassionate side of the unseen universal energy would be merciful to them.

After trying to bring up the subject of James with her father a couple of times at dinner or over a coffee and meeting extreme resistance, bordering on threats, Maria wasn't persuaded to stop seeing James. Contrary to her father's expectations she wanted to get to know him better but as James was a workaholic who didn't know what a weekend was, it was a challenge to find time together. He had given her a key to his new house and sometimes she would make an Italian dinner so that when he would arrive home after a fourteen-hour workday a nice meal would be waiting. They were growing closer and Maria was hoping they could find a normal balanced life together. Until then it was not clear if their romance was only an adventure of young love or something that could develop into a real relationship. They had talked seriously about living together, which was the obvious next step after months of dating. It would solidify their commitment and assure as much time together as possible. She had also gotten to know Greg better at the weekly yoga classes in James's living room. The advice he offered her was to be patient and not let go of James, who deep down was a person with a big heart but driven by hidden demons to prove something with his business. Greg also said James was no fool and really knew how precious Maria was. This gave her hope.

She finally was able to convince James to take an afternoon off and they drove in her car on some backcountry roads to the foothills above Saratoga and parked along the side of a one-lane road. They started following a dirt track that took them across open fields and through some apricot orchards. It eventually led to an expanse of vineyards and a distant small stone hut on a hill with an antique wine press and old oak barrels visible outside.

"I wanted to share this special place with you. It's my family's private retreat that only close friends know about," Maria said.

"I'm honored. It's magical up here. Like a step back in time."

"When I was growing up my father brought me here and shared stories about our family. He wanted me to understand the nobility of working with nature. He also taught me how to listen to the song of the earth. If you're really still you can hear the trees and grasses singing."

They stopped, quietly admiring the view. Slowly the sound of the wind in the trees and fields became more apparent accompanied by birdsong and buzzing bees.

Maria spoke softly, in awe of the nature. "Can you hear it?"

"It's one... it's all one..." James said softly having a momentary sensation of the connectedness he felt in India. After a minute of silent appreciation, he shared the story of the walk with the silent baba and discovering a similar oneness. Maria hugged him tight, feeling a special closeness beyond words.

They walked along the dirt road approaching the stone building. As they reached it, coming around the corner were surprised to see Maria's father sitting at a simple table with a glass of wine. He was as startled as them.

"Father," Maria said voicing her surprise.

Luigi looked at James with disdain knowing immediately who he was. "How dare you bring him here."

"It's alright – I consider James like family," Maria said.

"That's for to me to decide."

James started to speak. "Mr. Cappaletti—"

Luigi cut him off. "Listen, kid, I know who you are and if my daughter wasn't here I'd chew you up and spit you out."

"I know this isn't easy for you but we actually have a lot in common," James said.

"Like what – the death of my friend's son?"

"Sir, the police said the accident was his fault because he was legally drunk."

"That may be true. But I heard the whole shenanigans started because you wouldn't leave Maria alone." Luigi looked at James intently with piercing eyes.

"Tobias would have started a fight anyway. He was the type to think with his fists, not his brains," Maria said trying to find some middle ground.

Luigi looked at his daughter and replied with a hint of resignation, "You're right on that account. He was hotheaded and his father wasn't such a good influence. Is that what you two want to talk about?" He placed both hands flat on the table as if to restrain himself.

"Father, can we sit down and discuss this like grown-ups?"

"I suppose so," Luigi replied taking a long drink from his wine.

James pulled back a chair for Maria and then sat down and turned to face Luigi. "Thanks for the hospitality. I'd like to share my side of the story with you. You've built an empire of the best fruit orchards in the land and I'm also building something of value."

"Those nice words don't change the people who want to tear down my trees. I'd like to preserve something for future generations."

"Believe me, I completely sympathize with your situation but it's not as black and white as it seems."

Cappaletti paused, assessing James and said he knew the valley's history better than anyone. He offered his daughter and James a glass of wine that they accepted and he reluctantly clinked glasses with them. After James complimented Luigi on the vintage, he asked him about the family's history and the changing times. Mellowing more and more with each sip of wine, Mr. Cappaletti explained that the family had originally moved to the Santa Clara Valley when the repetitive farming of wheat in the 1800s had degraded the land and was replaced by fruit orchards. By the 1900s the area was full of orchards, and a couple of hundred fruit packing and drying companies with the Cappalettis leading the charge. There were scattered town centers like San Jose spread amongst the farms and the valley was relatively unspoiled. But with World War Two the young Luigi saw canning factories shifting their focus to supply war production. And after the war, as word got out about the mild climate and flat land that was easy to build on, the scattered city centers started to expand and the population grew steadily and eventually doubled just between 1950 and 1960. Suburbs grew with the blessings of the city councils eager to expand their tax base. Uncontrolled growth in housing and manufacturing sites for the newly developing electronics industry followed. The local politicians were in cahoots with developers who funded their election campaigns, built on a high growth platform.

Speculators offered farmers a couple of thousand dollars an acre that they gladly accepted when previously it had been valued at only five hundred an acre. A lot of farmers were already facing tearing up their hundred-year-old orchards to replant newer trees or else replace diseased trees damaged from a blight epidemic. This meant the farmers would have had to live off their savings until the new trees matured. But mostly it was the higher tax assessments after nearby lots sold to speculators at significantly higher prices that pressured them to sell. For the older families, inheritance taxes on the higher evaluations meant the land would have to pass out of the family ownership after it was resold to developers.

"This is fascinating so please excuse me for interrupting. I recall the farmers were able to lobby and get the county zoning laws changed to make certain areas exclusive for agriculture," James said.

"You're right but the city councils caved in to the developers, annexed the areas and took over zoning control where the developers wanted to build. And the best properties that would generate the most tax revenue were those designated for industrial plants." Luigi looked at James with a steady gaze and slowly took a swallow of wine.

"Mr. Cappaletti, I completely understand your situation."

"You have nothing to do with these new office complexes?"

"I started in my dad's garage building a dream and have had some modest success."

"And I read in the paper you want to change the world and are expanding your operations. I'm damn sure you can't do that without building more industry parks," Luigi said taking a gulp from his wine glass.

"Father, James spent a lot of time on a farm in Oregon, working in the apple orchards. He understands the nature of your business," Maria said.

Luigi gave James an appraising glance like there might be some hope for this technophile.

"I want to help folks enrich their lives by extending their natural capabilities. It's only when the people of this planet stop wanting what everyone else has and are happy with what they've got, will there be harmony," James said.

"You sure are idealistic, kid. And this…" Luigi made a sweeping gesture across the orchards including a construction crane in the distance. "See that building down there? It's sitting on land that used to be my best friend's orchards."

"There's no rule technology and farming can't coexist. I want to work with the farmers' coalition to find a more respectful approach," James said opening his arms expansively and carrying on with the gesture to swat at some pesky flies.

"And what? You'll join our protests and tell your friends to leave town?"

"Sir, if we can have a dialogue then we can find a way forward. Fighting won't change anything." James could see he was starting to gain some trust.

Luigi studied the young man, slowly getting convinced. "So, what's your plan then?"

"James has a lot of friends in the technology community. He can get them together to work with you and the other farmers," Maria said looking at her father intently.

Luigi paused thoughtfully then said reluctantly to James, "Okay, that's at least something." He rubbed his weathered hands over the table. "This table and chairs were made by my father out of the live oak from this hillside. He didn't use a single nail. Now everything is plastic from Japan."

"It's beautiful work," James said putting his hands on the table's surface.

"And your special gadgets – how do you plan on making enough of them to be a success?" Luigi asked pouring himself some more wine.

James knew he was skating on thin ice but had to say something, so he opted for the rational approach with a businesslike tact. "I'm investigating low-impact construction that is harmonious and respectful. My company just received a round of funding from a venture capital outfit named Kleiner-Perkins so we can hire good advisors—"

Luigi cut him off in a flash, his voice suddenly rising. "Those are the same bastards that funded Fairchild Semiconductor who tore down the best apricot orchards my family owned to make a chip plant." His voice was louder as the magic spell James had woven wore off. "You're as greedy as the worst of the lot."

"That was a different time—"

"And I suppose at the next city council meeting when they vote on zoning you will fight for the farmers." Luigi stood up and tossed his wine glass into the bushes. "I've tried to be a reasonable man. But if my daughter gets involved with someone I'd hope that if he didn't follow in our ways, he'd at least respect them." He disappeared into the small house, slamming the door.

Maria and James sat looking at each other not sure what to say or do next. James pushed his chair back from the table preparing to leave.

Maria had a sad expression and broke the silence

speaking quietly. "Why don't you let me talk to my dad once he's calmed down. I can catch a ride back with him."

"I guess that's the best way to handle it at this point. Go for it." James tried to sound upbeat but wasn't convincing.

"Thanks, darling. Here, take my car keys." Maria reached into her shoulder bag and found the keys, handing them to James. They both stood and James came around the table to share a quick kiss. "Call you later. Love you," Maria said softly.

"Love you too," James said with a smile, touching her shoulder. He walked slowly back down the trail through the vineyards, trying to make sense of what had just happened. He was wondering if Maria would end up taking her family's side and eventually abandon their relationship out of loyalty. He was starting to question where her allegiance really was. Perhaps abandoning a lifestyle she saw as a tradition and connection with more timeless values her family stubbornly tried to hold onto was really a possibility. Or maybe a happy medium could be found. On another level he was sure they both felt a deep connection as soul mates. Holding onto their past was a way to avoid entering something true that was beyond anything that had happened before and required giving up part of yourself. James knew there was little he could do to move closer to the farmers beyond what he had already done. He also believed in the valley as a home to greatness but with a more modern vision. The countryside was quiet as James followed the dirt path through the fields and the earth was still singing its song but James didn't hear it.

13

LILA MANDEVILLE AND THE YOGI OF THE STARS

Stephan sat in the reception area of a modest jewelry shop in Santa Monica on 4th Street by Wilshire waiting to get a new battery for his digital watch. He browsed a three-month-old city magazine while the owner of the shop was busy trying to pry the back off a crusty watch for an old lady. The ancient woman with pinkish hued silver hair was perched next to him grumbling with distrust in case the owner would try and switch watches if she took her eyes off him for one second. The bell attached to the shop door signaled a new customer. An attractive middle-aged lady, tastefully attired in a flower-print dress, came in with her daughter whose faded, painted-on jeans and belly-exposing T-shirt immediately caught Stephan's attention. The girl was about his age and a natural beauty, with luxurious dark hair curling to her shoulders and burning deep brown eyes. One glance from the shining angel made him momentarily forget his bearings. The mother chased down a couple of repairs from a Chinese clerk who looked like he had been working there since the original California gold rush. The daughter looked over at Stephan and smiled.

"Hi there, come to pick up the crown jewels?" Stephan inquired, taking advantage of the opening.

"Yes, there was a loose diamond in the royal scepter."

"My royal Seiko is also in need of attention." Stephan stood up slowly and held up his watch.

"Sounds like you're a busy man if you've run out of time," the young lady said, turning towards him with a pouting expression and a winking navel.

"I was told I could buy some here," Stephan said with a helpful smile leaning on the counter.

"I'll have to pick some up too."

"So, what's using up all your time these days?"

"I've got a role on a TV show and in-between learning the lines and getting the makeup put on my day just disappears."

"I know the routine. I've done some work lately on a comedy show, and it isn't all a bunch of laughs, as you know. I'm also taking some time to work with a partner on a publishing business. He has a place in Desert Hot Springs and I try to get out there and jump in the hot mineral water as much as I can to mellow out."

The girl reacted with a burst of enthusiasm like she had been offered an Oscar worthy script. "I go there all the time! I love to soak under the desert sky and watch the stars at night." Stephan was charmed by her natural Valley Girl phrasing that mashed up the R's and made half her sentences sound like questions.

That was enough of an introduction and they were immediately locked into an intense exchange on the virtues of curative waters in the healthy desert environment, combined with therapeutic yoga asanas. They would have jabbered away endlessly, but the girl's mother interrupted them politely indicating she had another errand. The woman had been watching Stephan out of the corner of her eye with the standard look of mistrust a mother has for fly-by-night suitors attracted by her daughter's good looks. The mother's accepted social protocol for making acquaintances was meeting over drinks at the Riviera Country Club. She looked at the two young people with a hint of a smile as she recognized there was something normal about their conversation compared to the usual Hollywood chatter.

Stephan asked the young lady if he could call her sometime to continue the conversation, and she happily agreed to meet for a coffee. She dug around in her purse and produced a card with a few makeup stains on it. Handing it to him, she announced her name was Lila, and Stephan then introduced himself with a firm handshake. Lila departed with her mother and Stephan shifted his focus to study the card where her name was printed across the middle in ornate Old English script: Lila Mandeville.

This being the city of image versus substance, Lila Mandeville was certainly not the lady's real name. It didn't surprise Stephan because even when a person talked like they were into an enlightened lifestyle, it was usually to compensate for being totally enmeshed in the world of superficiality. The next day they met for a cappuccino at an Italian diner in Westwood Village and with life being a perpetual audition, the actress made her story the center of the conversation.

The bar part of the restaurant was mostly empty before the lunchtime rush and Stephan had arrived early to find a free table. Lila was about ten minutes late and made a grand entrance with a scarf sailing behind her like she just finished an important meeting and was in a perpetual rush. Stephan stood and they did the European air kiss routine before sitting and complaining about the heat, Westwood parking and traffic on Wilshire. Stephan told her about some of the highlights from his short but eventful life that brought him to Los Angeles and the writing project he was working on.

"I suspected you were a fellow creative type. Do you think you can put the race in your story? Would make it really exciting."

"Great idea! Will have to see where I can fit it in."

She listened attentively to his Indian adventures which let her savor the feeling of being a seeker.

"That story of the girl and the fire is so intense. It's a bit too much to process right now, but I'm going to reflect on it and see what inner emotions it triggers. All part of learning a depth of emotion to help me in my roles." After they discussed the incident back and forth, she told Stephan her story with the usual fast-talking intensity.

"My mom used to be a casting agent. That was back when the studios were really studios and agents weren't so powerful. But that was twenty years ago, so a girls got to make her own way. I think success must be in the blood because here I am with a most divine role on a TV show."

"Hats off to you. I know it's very competitive being an actor. And nowadays it's even harder because the agents have all the power. The new breed all come with Harvard MBAs so it's all about product, not art."

"I figured the easiest way to break into the business was to start in TV, so I headed east and got a break acting in a soap opera. Maybe you heard of it – *General Hospital*." Stephan nodded sagely like he was a regular viewer.

"I am always amazed at how you can stand up in front of the camera day after day and do a scene like it's a nine-to-five job," Stephan said. The waitress appeared and put down a couple of glasses of ice water and took their order.

Lila made a confession. "Before I went to New York, I changed my name to something more artistic and original to help me stick out from the crowd."

"Not to mention, look good up on a marquee."

"That's right, it's very important." She took a quick sip of water and continued her tale. "My real name is Jane Black, which isn't the ticket to a starring role. Boring with a large capital 'B'. My parents weren't thinking of an acting career for me when they dreamed that one up." They both laughed. "I decided to call myself Lila. It's the Hindu word meaning divine play, the endless dance of life that God observes with a watchful grin. And Mandeville sounded classy and British. Besides, the letters added up to a favorable combination, according to the numerology expert I consulted."

Lila did well enough to become a regular on the soap opera hospital tearjerker for a couple of years. After a succession of boyfriends and a healthy dose of New York angst, neurosis and street mania, decided she was ready to go for the big time in Los Angeles and move up from video to celluloid film. Lila showed Stephan one of her composite photos that she routinely left with producers, and it reminded him of the ones on the walls in Malone's office. In the main photo of her in a chic evening gown, she looked as elegant as any high-class lady in a European grand casino and the smaller shot of her in a bikini with a petulant look promised pleasures that could make a grown man go weak in the knees.

Lila explained she kept herself in shape and her energy at a high level from yoga classes with an Indian yoga teacher named Bilkem. His style of hot yoga attracted some Hollywood A-list clients and gave impressive results. She was a regular student and also working on a yoga teaching degree. Stephan agreed to go with her the next day. Lila encouraged Stephan to join in because of all the benefits she found like flexibility, strength, inner poise and an ass you could bounce quarters off.

The students gathered in a remodeled office space above a Chinese restaurant south of Sunset, packed in like cars in a shopping mall parking lot at Christmas. One additional benefit that Stephan discovered in the class was more eye candy per square foot than he could imagine finding even at the Playboy mansion. Most ladies were like Lila, aspiring actresses where their body was their tool of commerce. Tight buns, firm breasts and a narrow waist could get an audition faster than a résumé of sold-out performances with the Royal Shakespeare Company. This wasn't the laid-back relaxing school of yoga where a gentle stretch was backed up by philosophy and affirmations that calmed the mind like Stephan and Greasy used to teach. This was all-out bone crunching gymnastics, aimed at creating the curves and flat planes the customers desired. Nothing was without its price, and the twenty dollars a lesson, long lines of willing supplicants and high-priced private sessions assured that Bilkem had a couple of Bentleys plus a penthouse in an apartment tower on an upmarket stretch of Wilshire. All to help with his Western-style ascetic monk's life.

Bilkem had quickly realized that the public in America responded well to a Marine Corps drill sergeant routine and barked out orders in-between name-dropping the times he spent with Elvis, the pope and one of the Beatles. Stephan was already sweating profusely ten minutes into the class and while the positions weren't too difficult the 102-degree heat made it a challenge. With only a towel to lie on he noticed the industrial carpeting was giving off a locker-room funk like unwashed gym shorts from all the sweat it had absorbed over the months. The class had only about thirty people so Bilkem could zero in on individual students with a mix of criticism and praise pushing people to go an extra inch.

Stephan liked the classes and enjoyed getting to know Lila better but after a couple of dinners and no more than a brotherly hug at the end it dawned on him it was the same scene that had unfolded earlier with Greg and his actress friend. Men in this town were only useful if they had the connections to get you in a movie or else support a lifestyle that made acting a luxury. He had hoped that with their mutual interests and creative backgrounds he had discovered his muse who not only would inspire and support him but was somehow also respectful of the inner path he was pursuing. He remembered Greg's words when they parted about keeping the focus in the midst of the illusion. Stephan thought having a partner who could see the inner and outer worlds like he did would be the key. He let his fantasies take flight imagining the two of them opening a yoga center in the desert once Lila had her teaching degree.

They hadn't seen each other for a few weeks and then one night after meeting up for a yoga class they went to dinner. As was their routine, they went to the Good Earth restaurant in Westwood, to supplement the vital energy called prana that their feverish exertions generated. They ordered the standard meal of organic carrot juice and a sandwich with unknown mushy vegetables topped with the requisite alfalfa sprouts on stone ground bread with many unidentifiable tasteless crunchy bits.

They were sitting at a booth near the door so Lila could catch the eye of any possible studio executives. She whispered to Stephan, "Let me know if the waitress is looking." In her local dialect it sounded like she was asking him a question. When Stephan gave a coast-is-clear signal, Lila deftly slipped the jar of Dijon mustard from the condiments tray into her purse. While she sported the look of success, she had the budget of a starving artist that meant she routinely purloined the organic salt and herb shakers from the tabletop. Stephan knew that Lila had burned her way through a lot of her savings in pursuit of stardom, and was considering selling her stake in a condo that her accountant had put Lila's soap money into as a tax shelter.

"I sure hope I can make the break into film from TV because if you get type-cast as a TV actress it's hard to get considered for real roles. I've gone on three auditions this week but no callbacks. My agent says to be patient but I'm almost twenty-five."

"Don't worry, you look like you're still eighteen. I think all that yoga is the secret of eternal youth."

"You're so sweet. I may not be stunning but I have character." She blew him an air kiss.

Stephan was momentarily distracted watching the waitress serve some good smelling veggie burgers to the next table. "What's more you have an inner fire which people can feel. I know that side of you because we have a similar direction in life. Even someone like an agent must sense that potential. Few people can offer that extra dimension."

"Most of these producers are such lowlifes. It's not in their realm of capability to recognize something on that level." She paused to take a sip from her juice and scan the people coming and going. "I'm tired of the small jobs but I need to keep my résumé fresh with new roles or else I look undesirable. Last week it was a TV ad for folding bicycles and a milk commercial. My last real role was on a two-bit Western and even that was as an extra." Lila looked around at the other diners in case any of them were listening.

"I really admire your work ethic. You're the hardest working lady in Hollywood," Stephan said raising his glass in a mock toast.

"You said it. I spend hours preparing for the interviews, getting the makeup just right and my hair. Always need the tightest pair of jeans and no undies in case the producer sees a VPL," Lila said brightly like she was being interviewed on network television.

"A what?" Stephan asked through a mouthful of sandwich.

"Visible panty line. Only grandmothers wear saggy panties under their jeans. And then when I'm tarted up the producer thinks it's an invite to stick his hand in my jeans like one did last week. The guy thought I must be desperate." The last line sounded like a question. "But anyway, it did get me a role as a nurse on a *CHiPs* episode." She went back to work on her sandwich cutting it into bite-sized pieces.

"What a creep. Let me know when I can see you on TV."

"My real highlight last week was going to a party where Clint Eastwood was a guest. I maneuvered through his entourage and sat on his knee like he was my sugar daddy. I knew he was casting for his next film but that bastard gave the role to his horse-faced girlfriend the next day."

"You really did that? You're amazing!" Lila smiled and tossed her hair over her shoulder like such actions were just part of the job.

In spite of her ambitions and frustrations she had a heart of gold when the dust of seeking fame didn't tarnish it. Stephan took the opportunity of their evolved plutonic friendship to share an update on his novel and casually pitched his story to Lila as a potential starring vehicle. She particularly liked the idea if she could play the goddess role and said she would talk it up wherever she could.

Lila was inspired to help Stephan as much as she was interested to be seen on the arm of a cute young guy. When she called him again a couple of days later to escort her to a film screening, Stephan thought at first that she had come to realize the quality of their relationship and that they were meant to be partners. She explained it was a private screening at a major studio so a lot of executives would be there and she needed an attractive date. She hadn't meant the comment to put him down but rather cast him as a good-looking hunk, but Stephan nevertheless was hurt. He felt he was being used and all their time together was looking like he had been providing emotional support to a fragile actress's ego and their relationship might be just one more role Lila was playing. He felt naïve and remembered some words from the silent baba: 'attachment is blinding and lends an imaginary halo of attractiveness to the object of desire'.

Stephan liked to think he was developing a more serious attitude towards the opposite sex that was more focused on having a respectful relationship rather than the more enjoy-it-while-you-can attitude he had learned from Greg. He also knew that Lila did like him and could see they were suited for each other. It was clearly obvious as she hadn't found something that good anywhere else until now. He reminded himself that relationships could be a waiting game and if they could be friends, the door would always be open to take the next step. But it was certainly frustrating to be around this woman at times. Stephan begged off, complaining he had another engagement and decided to manage his enthusiasm and pull back from an active pursuit.

Lila had sensed his cooling-off towards her and she called a few days later to give him an update on the screening and announce she had finally landed a role in a film. She shared the exciting news like she would with any good friend. She explained a British director had been in town casting for a remake of a Charles Bronson revenge film and after a dinner with him at his Beverly Hills villa he was convinced she should play the role of the supporting actress. They were going to Santa Barbara for the weekend to discuss the script. Filming would start in a couple of weeks, spanning the next two months. Stephan wanted to feel good about Lila getting the role as he knew she was talented and deserved a break but he also felt she was selling herself out knowing that the clock was ticking. Meanwhile she was getting the best of both worlds – career advancement and a well-matched guy hanging around to fill in any gaps. A part of him was also a bit jealous because the life he had imagined for them was being lived by someone else.

It might have been consoling for Stephan to know that Lila, for all her fast talking and bright personality, subconsciously knew because of the contrast he provided that her moral bank account was being chipped away by all the casual arrangements that were easy to fall into in the name of networking and acting out the role of a much-desired diva.

14

MONEY IS THE ROOT OF ALL GOOD

Maria maintained a form of détente with her parents, based on an 'ask me no questions and I'll tell you no lies' policy. She did this to try and dance between the issues of maintaining her closeness to her family while growing into a new life of her own. She had her small and large battles with them over James and in the end started spending more nights at James's home than her parents', which helped him believe that she had found the balance between her two worlds. She was twenty-two, which made her legally an adult, so while her parents' influence was limited they used every opportunity and means possible to make her see their point of view.

Maria did her best to fix up the old Victorian James had acquired in Los Gatos, but as could be expected he had some strong ideas about how he wanted it decorated. James had moved from his Indian influenced yogi days to a more modern, twentieth-century belief in Zen Buddhism's Japanese minimalist look. The India print bedspreads that had hung on the walls, altars with pictures of saints and Hindu statues, with an ever-present smell of incense had disappeared. In their place, a sleeker modern look of bare simplicity and stylized Asian dark wood and chrome furniture appeared.

This change of lifestyle was fueled in part by James's sense of frustration from his failed dreams of finding a teacher in India to show him an inner reality and witnessing a traditional ceremony that disqualified any holy beliefs he may have adopted. When the trip's outcome didn't match his desired framework of well-defined results he could control, and the business demands were turning his life into a pressure cooker, he decided to embrace another variety of the path to enlightenment – the study of Zen Buddhism. This school of thought focused on the same inner goal, but with techniques that better matched his ever more modern life that mixed his spiritual aspirations with yet another healthy diet with strict rules. Gone were the raw-food regimes and lacto-ovo vegetarianism, and in their place was macrobiotics as a way of balancing the yin and yang. Achieving higher consciousness through tofu. This meant rice and miso every day with some wakame and kuzu enhanced seaweed on black beans and even sushi became acceptable. Buckwheat pasta placated Maria's Italian cravings at the frequent late-night dinners they shared, even though she took to lunchtime binges at the university's cafeteria or a local eatery on University Avenue for a real burger and fries.

Maria rose to the challenge of James's Eastern views, while her tastes tended to a sunnier Mediterranean style. Participating in the decorating, she was able to work out compromises so some of her original art could be hung in the house, and the kitchen was designed with a rustic wooden style and hanging copper pots like a Tuscan farmer's kitchen. She was still painting at Montalvo while finishing her studies at Stanford. Her parents hoped that by attending classes she would gradually move in other circles and perhaps meet a nice Italian boy whose background more matched their own.

James came home early one Friday afternoon and kidnapped Maria in his bus to spend a long weekend together. They had a leisurely drive along the coast to Big Sur, visiting the many rustic art galleries scattered above the wild dramatic shoreline. James stopped frequently for them to admire the views along Highway 1 where it daringly snaked around over steep cliffs that dropped straight into a vibrant blue sea, framed with a border of white sand beaches. James would explain local mythology that included the claim that the area was a lost Japanese island joined with the mainland, which is why its unique geography and vegetation mirrored the distant lands.

Acting like natives they ran naked on remote beaches, diving into the cold, crystalline water and stayed the night at a mountaintop Zen center. There they soaked in natural mineral water baths, while looking over the rolling hills and endless ocean and enjoyed the fresh bread prepared by Zen monks. For a real adventure in nature, they hiked with backpacks up the Big Sur River and camped overnight at some remote hot springs above the riverbank that was a favorite location for itinerant travelers. While hiking, James would scare Maria by tossing stones into old cisterns along the trail, and the angry buzzing of a handful of trapped rattlesnakes would remind her of the wild nature of the land. Maria endlessly sketched the unique perspectives of the dramatic gorge while James would quietly contemplate Buddhist literature. He was seeking clues to a moment of satori, where the underlying Buddha nature of the universe would be revealed. They felt removed from the modern world as the gently rolling river, spilling over water-worn rocks harmonized with the stillness of the remote location. The two days of adventure and simple living brought them closer than they had ever felt possible, bringing their relationship to a new level.

While James would host dinners at the house to meet Maria's circle of friends, he also supported Maria in organizing yoga classes with Greg for her girlfriends in the living room. He and Greg had an awkward friendship with each too proud to find a way to put the race behind them. James had compartmentalized it by bringing his focus exclusively on the business and when time allowed, Maria. The world seemed to be moving on so the rap sessions he used to have with Greg that tried to solve the world's problems were as outdated as the Homebrew Computer Club. To make an attempt at maintaining their connection, James had offered Greg the use of his home. James never attended any of the classes so the news he got about Greg was always secondhand, relayed by Maria. She and Greg had been able to make a diplomatic peace over the racing tragedy after many long discussions; and perhaps James felt that Maria's friendly connection covered him so no more effort was required on his part to resolve any unspoken issues.

To prepare for the classes Maria would move the furniture aside and Greg would arrive in full yogi attire, beaming a benevolent smile at the sight of a half dozen young ladies, waiting for the wise and caring teacher from afar to dispense his pearls of wisdom. At the end of the session everyone received a mild neck massage while lying flat on their backs in the corpse posture. Afterwards, Greg would entertain his admiring audience with imitations of everyone from a ghetto brother to a noble yogi whose righteous words were mixed with his material desires. He would slip in a few snippets of wisdom he had interpreted in his own way to show that stretching was only one small step on the way to the place of contentment everyone had inside. Greg would flirt outrageously, making each lady feel they were his sole interest and a bright shining star while assigning each student a pet name like 'babe-a-lino' for Maria's cousin Gloria from Santa Cruz. Maria knew Greg and her cousin would meet occasionally for lunch by the beach but neither of them was forthcoming with Maria as to the extent of their relationship. It was understood that what happens in Santa Cruz stays in Santa Cruz. But Maria hoped Gloria, who was a teacher's assistant in the English department at the university, could provide some grounding energy for Greg.

Maria won over the hearts of the crew at James's office by baking up huge piles of chocolate-chip cookies and delivering them with her girlfriends, causing a welcome distraction for the dedicated engineers. The technically focused staff didn't know which was more uplifting, the sugar high or the cute ladies dispensing the goodies to the usual all-male enclave. James graciously accepted the interruptions, and even Grok would leave his office to join in the impromptu coffee break, insisting Maria make him a real Italian espresso. The Garden of Eden was the Biblical representation of heaven on earth, but even with Maria's welcome distractions James was gradually helping Eden Computers turn into the personification of a living hell. It wasn't by plan that this was meant to happen. Eve had never planned for her and a dude named Adam to get tossed out of an idyllic garden because of snacking on a biologically grown, pesticide-free piece of fruit offered by a friendly reptile, which was being helpful by interpreting the big boss's intent.

James had a dream and as is typical with visionaries, believed nobody else could understand or attain his ideal of perfection. In his eyes, neither the engineers working day and night building innovative features nor the president driving sales through the roof could fully grasp his same unique vision. There was a sense of impatience and restlessness, which was deep down inside ultimately fear-driven. The angst that someone would develop a faster, cooler box and make the Eden machines irrelevant. The computer for the masses had been James's vision and he wanted to see it realized, but time waited for nobody, not even visionaries. The credit went to the winners, not the losers.

With James's single-pointed drive, Eden was fantastically successful beyond anyone's wildest imagination with their latest model, the Eden II. There was competition appearing but nobody could match the ease of use and stylish designs his devices offered. The talk now was to go on the New York Stock Exchange and be the fastest company to hit the Fortune 500 rankings. As founders and majority shareholders, James and Grok had become millionaires without even trying and their earnings until now would pale by what they would receive from exercising their stock options. You wouldn't know it to look at them in their typical office attire.

One of the biggest battles that rocked the firm started between the normally laid-back Grok and the hard-charging James, over Grok's role in the future of the company. Grok had wanted to retire and tinker with designs for innovative gizmos, while James knew Grok's engineering genius would define the success of the future models. James had tried his hand at designing a new machine but it ended up not being as functional or easy to use as he imagined. Hundreds of thousands spent in development costs for features that sounded cool but couldn't practically be delivered into a commercial machine were the end result.

The fun was out of the game for Grok now that it was a mass-market business and not a small group of individuals with a unique hobby, each trying to be a better hacker than the other. The next challenges were unknown, but with the luxury of not having to worry about earning a salary, he could pursue any idea that suited his fertile imagination.

Compounding the mix of problems to propel him out of the company, was Grok finally learning a well-hidden secret of when James ripped him off for doing some engineering work at Atari. One of the older engineers on the programming team, who had once freelanced at Atari, accidentally mentioned the incident when Grok was around. While an employee of the games company, James had been asked to design a new chip to power a next-generation arcade game. He knew Grok was better at engineering and asked for his help, knowing Grok loved a challenge more than the financial reward. The deal would pay more when fewer transistors were required in the design, so while quoting Grok a flat rate of a few hundred dollars, James was actually paid several thousand. He'd been trying to get money together to buy into an Oregon commune and was able to motivate Grok with the challenge of merely reducing the number of transistors in the design.

When Grok confronted him, James was defensive at first, saying not to worry because it was only money and now they each had more than they knew what to do with. After a pause where Grok stared at James with a mix of disappointment and skepticism, James apologized, citing their friendship as being more valuable than money and acknowledged that he had been out of line. He said he had been a different person back then and it was better to leave the past in the past and look forward.

Grok wasn't placated in his anger and stormed out of the office and didn't return any calls. Instead of being able to try and squeeze more time out of his heavy schedule for Maria, James had to spend extra hours in the office, maintaining the engineering department to keep development schedules on time. In a late-night meeting with the programmers they discussed various options to avoid any slippage in the roadmap that would delay key features and cause a ripple effect on other elements being designed. James worked on playing down their fears, as there had been an added sense of urgency to their planning because they all knew the competition wasn't sleeping. IBM's announcement of their own type of personal computer was the biggest threat, because when the world's largest computer company jumps into a market, there are bound to be waves.

The bigger mountain on the horizon to scale was the pending IPO. It had been built up with the original venture capital firm and an investment bank paving the way to going on the Big Board – the NYSE. The deal was pretty much wrapped up with all the shareholders making profits on their options, with the two founders at the fixing looking to be double-digit millionaires in their early twenties. Grok's absence from the investor briefings didn't help, which made the management team scramble more than usual, but there was enough forward momentum to carry on regardless. Grok wasn't impressed with the upcoming listing and was talking about opening his own lab and wanting to put on some large concerts that introduced friendly technology to teenagers.

It wasn't a surprise when Grok formally took an open-ended sabbatical a couple of weeks later and the engineering team lost an ally on the management board. James then had open season on cajoling, brow beating and shouting to get results, without the buffer of Grok to shield the engineers. It was like Grok had served as his conscience. Without that presence, the more negative demanding aspects of James's personality that had been held in check, could now run free with the stress factor amplifying them more than normal. When it came to engineering, James always got involved in every discussion about transistors and schematics, reviewing prototype boards wanting everything perfect down to the smallest detail and also coached the engineers to help raise the level of their work.

To add to the stress, Mike Markulla, the seed investor who got Eden off the ground, was making demands and had installed at his insistence a president who challenged James on several occasions about marketing and development issues, and another power struggle broke out. James wanted to be everything for everybody at the company, micromanaging every area, including the business side. While a ruthless negotiator when it came to grinding suppliers, all sense of compromise was lost in debates over running the company.

One morning when James was having a meeting in a conference room with Markulla and the president, an older industry veteran, the conversation got heated, bordering on an outright argument. The president had wanted to introduce some features which market research had said would make the computers more interesting for consumers and therefore signal the investors that the company was really mainstream-focused, not a company for elite hobbyists. They cited the example of a rival company called Commodore who had just announced a low-priced computer and were aiming for a mass-market product. James argued that he knew the industry and market better than anyone and therefore knew what was best for the company. He had started the outfit and created the original vision that he felt was important to the long-term direction they should aim for. The president wouldn't back down and James stood up to make his point while the two older executives sat patiently at the large meeting table watching the performance of James pacing back and forth making his case. There was no compromise from either side and James raised the stakes by threatening to resign, with the argument ending when James walked out. Markulla escalated the issue to the board and in a similarly acrimonious session the board sided with the president and James gave up the fight. The tension was released for the moment, but a sense of dissatisfaction remained on both sides.

But now it looked like the honeymoon was over both professionally and privately. James was late getting home as was becoming the standard routine and being so wound up from the day, he bounced off the walls for an hour, blasting Bob Dylan's poetry in motion, *Blood on the Tracks*, over his monster stereo system while quickly downing some rice and beans with a glass of red wine. Watching him so stressed out, the old doubts Maria had would resurface and she would wonder what she had gotten herself into. It was her first real relationship and their living arrangement meant that she had occasional nights at her parents' house where the low-key suburban world seemed more normal at times than her new life at the moment. While she busied herself in the kitchen the words from the song 'Shelter from the Storm' playing in the background echoed her mood:

Now there's a wall between us, somethin' there's been lost

I took too much for granted, got my signals crossed
Just to think that it all began on a non-eventful morn

"Come in," she said, "I'll give you shelter from the storm."

Finally, James slowed down enough that they could find their moment of bonding and they curled up together on the sofa exchanging stories from their day's events. She told him he should relax but there was an underlying sense of James not being content. Maria explained she had arranged for Greasy to come over for dinner and received an indifferent grunt for a reply. She hoped Greg's jive talking and free and easy lifestyle would be a momentary reminder of the not so long ago good old days and a subliminal message to James that it was okay to relax. It was her attempt at bridging the gap between James's past and present, with some distant hopes of reviving a softer James.

Greg had been showing up every couple of weeks in-between the yoga classes, whether James was there or not. They all knew James felt completely safe being able to trust Maria and Greg together, in spite of Greg's reputation in tantric yoga. Greg worshipped Maria and treated her like royalty. Especially because she would offer him ciabatta sandwiches for lunch, as Los Gatos was on the way back over the hill to Santa Cruz from his driving trips around the Bay Area. But in spite of all the efforts on Greg's part to establish a cozy connection with Maria, she had a cool and detached side to her Greg could not entirely break through. It became a challenge for Greg to win her over as he was used to women being immediately charmed by his antics and insightful words. And the fact she wasn't so easily swayed made her special because it was only by honestly sharing his deeper feelings and expressing his emotions that he could hope to bond with this lady.

While Maria liked Greg, it was a bit difficult for her at times to speak with him knowing that he was directly involved with her friend's death. Every time they would meet there was always a touch of sadness mixed with a portion of anger. She really enjoyed Greg's company but her feelings of the unnecessary death never really went away. In their lunch meetings Greg would give her tips on how to manage James, having known him for many years as well as sharing secrets from the male-female dynamics he had learned from his many encounters with ladies. Maria would listen but there was always a sense his words were being heard with a critical ear. And when Greg confessed to still feeling guilty about Tobias's death Maria assured him it really wasn't all his fault. She also pointed out that having a deadly race over a girl trivialized the sanctity of life, by reducing it to a sporting event. Greg had no answer to the accusation, so the rightful anger Maria felt hung in the air.

The room had quieted after the last comment and then Greg added, "You know what scares me the most?" He paused and looked her square in the eyes. "That to bury my guilt, I need chemical help to make the memory livable."

Maria responded, "Why is it always about you? Nobody you were close to died and now you're back zooming down the highways like nothing happened." Greg looked away with a sad expression, staring out the kitchen window to the backyard in a rare moment of not being sure what to say next. She watched him a second and suddenly it dawned on her what he meant. All the cravings for sweets and extended bathroom visits made sense now. A sense of fear rose up inside her, perhaps from sensing another potential death in her circle of friends. Her tone changed immediately to one of caring. "Oh no, Greg, please don't do what I think you mean. Your heart is too good and you have so much to offer than to go down that path. Be strong." She put her hand on his forearm where they sat at the kitchen table. Greg placed his hand on top of hers and thanked her. Maria wasn't convinced her words would have much influence and she inwardly said a prayer for his overcoming any obstacles.

She masked her judgmental feelings and hoped as time passed she could fully let go of them and see Greg as just another friend of James. She wondered if that day would ever come as he tried to be a good buddy she could share her heart with. Greg knew James and all his sides and was deep down an innocent soul with simple life-wisdom to share.

The night of the dinner, Greg was late as usual, and James had gotten bombed on some macrobiotic beer from Boston. He had already started eyeing the saki he was going to uncork for dinner, when Greg roared into the drive with his latest vintage Porsche. He popped out of the car striding up the drive with "howdies" and "what's up" tossed out before clenching Maria and laying a loud smacking kiss on her cheek with a: "You're looking fine, mama," in his best pimp-on-the-street twang to complement the physical appreciation. James was smiling, because Greg's jokes always put him in a good mood. He was a fellow dharma bum looking for enlightenment, albeit in a more unconventional manner, but a seeker of deeper meanings nonetheless.

"How's it hanging, big guy?" Greg said to James, punching him playfully in the arm.

"Fine. Everything's fine, just keep on keeping on," James replied quoting Dylan, feeling a bit loose from the beer.

"Right on, brother. Gimme five. Slip me some change." They slapped hands. "That's right, be cool."

They moved into the living room and Greg gladly accepted a beer from Maria and paced around tinkering with the stereo controls, too restless to sit still. He flipped through the stack of albums and pulled out one by Led Zeppelin and set the needle down on their FM radio classic, 'Stairway to Heaven'. He cranked the volume up and started an improvised Kathak Indian temple dance with hand mudras and spastic leg movements. Then he broke into playing an invisible guitar, to copy the solo that was meant to transport the listener to a higher dimension. He turned the volume down before the end of the song and went back to inspecting the record collection. James and Maria watched from the low futon sofa and when the music was quieter after Greg put on *Songs in the Key of Life*, they talked about the remodeling underway. As they spoke Greg inventoried the décor curious about each Japanese brushstroke's symbology and even more curious about the recent paintings Maria had created.

They all found their way to the table balancing on round cushions, atop tatami mats that covered the dining room floor. The long, wide table was black lacquer and low to the ground. When the traditional Japanese meal was artistically presented, Greg twirled his chopsticks like a cheerleader with a baton, in-between fiddling with the stringy seaweed.

"Sure is better than that fruit diet you were always on. At least there's some bulk here," Greg commented. There were piles of brown rice, black beans, sushi, exotic vegetable tempura, miso soup and corn bread. Maria was an excellent cook and had picked up on the Japanese menu quickly.

The talk at dinner was mostly James going on about his business expansion and how much money they were making. Greg countered with, "And so money is the root of all good then?" and carrying on with the usual elaborate descriptions of wild parties at the Catalyst saloon in Santa Cruz and endless car stories.

Greg changed the direction of the conversation and stood up to act out a party scene he was detailing to the embarrassment of James. "Then James tried to get out the front door but he was so blitzed on beer he was walking sideways like a crab and couldn't find the door handle because his back was facing it." Greg feigned a groping James to everyone's amusement. "But of course, we made him sit it out until he could touch his nose while standing on one foot."

"I seem to remember even you, the great yogi, would take an hour to conquer that pose on a good night without any drinks," James replied as everyone laughed some more.

"Those were formative years to be sure," Greg said.

"We moved on to all-night meditation sessions or doing shaman ceremonies watching fluorescent plankton on the cosmic beach we called 'hole in the wall' because it had this amazing natural arch."

"Those sure were simpler times when enchantment and timelessness were our normal existence," James said wistfully, leaning back and taking a sip of green tea from his rough ceramic mug.

"Yeah, there was always this childlike sense of possibility and wonder," Greg added sitting down again.

Maria broke the quiet that developed as the two friends smiled at each other sharing a telepathic memory of a magical time. "Any stories of James's past conquests I should know about?"

James shook his head emphatically in a 'no' motion begging that no secrets be shared so Greg told about James getting so drunk in the redwoods that he woke up without knowing a giant electric yellow banana slug had crawled across his face, leaving a fat dry trail of slime for the others to admire.

Maria started to tell a few stories of her own about some of the wild parties she went to in high school when parents left their houses to wayward girls for the weekend, only to return to trashed living rooms with empty beer cans turning up in every corner and severely hung-over teenagers sleeping in the laundry room.

They were all laughing at their stupidity, each trying to show they were the silliest but at the end of the party after the plum ice-cream and green tea the mood changed. James announced his latest purchase of a 1950s Mercedes and his intent to take some professional driving lessons so he could enter the annual classic car race in Monterey. Greg mumbled some words that were meant to sound like an upbeat compliment, but they mostly faded before reaching anyone's ears. He felt James was trying to rub success in his face while also saying that he could manage to race a car successfully as if it were something one could learn in a weekend course.

Greg looked at Maria to change the subject and said, "Hey, baby, what's goin' on," like he was a soul brother talking to his soul sister. He got up to fiddle some more with the stereo and announced he was leaving. The two hosts stood up and Greg said his goodbyes to Maria with a sexy squeeze and thanked her for the meal. He added that if she weren't hooked up with James, he would surely steal her away. She gave him a quick peck on the cheek and said he should keep his eyes on the road.

Greg and James went out through the garage to see James's newest toy. Greg unlatched the hood, lifted the cover and momentarily inspected the classic Mercedes engine with a few approving 'hmms' before sitting in the driver's seat to check out the controls. Feeling a moment of camaraderie James took the opportunity to tell a Zen story about two monks that illustrated how to let go of negative thoughts that had become habit. Greg listened patiently and although it was James's way of suggesting that Greg move on from his guilt from the race and resulting actions, it came out more like a lecture. Greg responded that such serious incidents weren't easily forgotten and reminded James how he always referred back to the fire ceremony he had witnessed in India as a reminder of the mystery of life and death. Greg thought James should be taking counsel from his own words, as the subject of the race hadn't been brought up, as it was still awkward for James to discuss it. He then explained how yoga also taught flexibility of thinking as well as the body and asked if he knew that Abraham was the most flexible man in the Bible.

"No, I didn't."

"He was so flexible, that he could tie his ass to a tree and walk all the way to Jericho," Greg said with a flourish.

James laughed for a moment and started back on the merits of his car, as if Greg's words weren't meant for him. With James's incessant chattering about all the marvels of his car, Greg who was an already annoyed mechanic frustrated with the one-way dialogue, had finally lost his cool. He was now angry at James's showing off again and ignoring the issue at the heart of their relationship.

Greg climbed out of the Benz and slammed the door unnecessarily hard. James started to say something about respecting the car but Greg turned his back and walked determinedly out the open garage door to his Porsche with his head down, watching the ground. He got in, banged the door closed and started the motor with a loud roar. He waved goodbye by flashing a quick peace sign as he backed down the drive. As he entered the street he turned and pointed the car down the lane, grabbed the steering wheel with one hand and jammed the stick shift into first gear. He started revving the engine so that when he released the clutch he left a ten-foot long strip of burnt rubber on the road.

Maria watched from the window smoking a cigarette and when James came in she extinguished it in an ashtray, crossed the room and sat cross-legged on the futon sofa asking him to join her.

"What is Greg angry about, I thought you two were friends?"

"I guess he can't accept that I've made something of my life and he's still trying to find a purpose," James said taking a pull from a beer he had picked up in the kitchen.

"But he's happy with his life – isn't that enough? Weren't you the first to say that peace of mind and fulfillment isn't about how much you've got, but if you have contentment?" She was watching him as he stared ahead, looking out the window at the rock garden in the backyard.

"True, but if you don't do something to share your understanding, then what's the use. If I don't try and help the world with tools to support a humanitarian vision, then I might as well go live in a monastery or a cave in the mountains." He repositioned himself on the sofa to look her in the eyes.

"All I see is bigger, better, faster. Sure, you have a dream with Eden, but you can't forget those people close to you. Greg's a dear friend and now you've totally alienated him. And sometimes I feel that I'm your one-person missionary project of converting me to your concept of a healthy life and inner peace. But guess what – I'm a feeling person, not an intellectual. Or maybe I'm just another finished project and now you can focus on your business."

"I'm sorry; I thought we were coming closer together by spending more time with each other. And it's not my wish to convert you to any exclusive worldview." James reached over and put his hand gently on her shoulder until her chilly look made him remove it.

"You've made Eden into a cause as big as any religious movement on the planet, but at what price? One of your best friends just left here totally pissed-off because you didn't see behind his words he's calling for help. And I'm starting to feel the same way." Her voice broke at the end as if she was going to cry and she lowered her head blinking back tears.

James got up and started pacing. "Wait a minute. Yes, Greg is no doubt a brother and we've shared a lot of life experiences but I don't owe him anything and he doesn't owe me anything." He stopped his pacing with his back to the window and turned to her with a hand on his hip and the other by his side holding the beer. "For sure we're still friends but he's got his life and I've got mine. And if they diverge in different directions, then that's the evolution of personal growth."

"Maybe you should finally wake up and see what individual development really is. If your eyes were even halfway open like you imagine they are you would have seen Greg is strung out on God knows what – probably heroin. But instead of doing something to help him with a bit of your so-called Buddhist compassion, you're letting him fall deeper into his hell. Maybe even pushing him faster along that road." Maria's voice was rising and she punched a pillow next to her to emphasize her point.

"He's been around long enough to know how to deal with issues."

"And me? Is my dissatisfaction my own problem? I thought we were in this together. Isn't that what a loving partnership is all about?" Maria said.

James resumed his pacing and paused facing her from next to the fireplace. "No doubt about it. I hear you and it's important to understand I also have other priorities."

"So where am I on the list? Position five?" She glared at him a second to let her point to sink in. "I think your problem is you have some kind of hidden frustration of being in Greg's debt and it should have been you in the car that night. Racing your old Mercedes is not going to get rid of the guilt. And because you can't let go of it and move on you're starting to look as pigheaded as my parents. Who, in case you hadn't noticed, hate you more than ever, especially after that chat with my dad. I think you even feel guilty about loving me, because if we hadn't met this whole race story wouldn't have happened."

James took a last final swill to finish his beer and moved to the window staring at an invisible distant horizon, one arm against the window frame, the other by his side holding the empty bottle. He spoke to the dark garden, "We at least have each other and I thought at the end of the day that is what really mattered."

"That was how we started but now that connection looks like it is starting to fade," Maria said in a sad tone.

He turned his head to look at her. "I'm sorry. Please try and understand my situation. I know we can find a way forward."

"Between Eden and your issues with the race there's not much space left for me."

"What are you talking about? I'm here for you," James said turning fully to face her.

Maria was crying now and stood up, moving in front of James. As he looked at her she swung her open hand, striking him across the cheek.

"What's that?" James said, surprised.

"An answer to the old Zen question – what's the sound of one hand clapping." She stomped out of the room, slamming the bedroom door behind her.

James was initially stunned. He would never have expected such a reaction, thinking all was cool and under control. That momentary ego wave of self-importance faded and, in its place, came a temporary state of no-mind awareness. The rug had been pulled out from underneath him and all that he believed to be true was momentarily suspended.

James was aware of the tingling of the skin on his cheek and the echo of the slap still rang in his ears. He used his mindfulness training to stay with the moment and not be distracted. His breathing quieted and an unexpected feeling of compassion welled up inside. He decided against going back to the office and went out to the garden and sat on a small bench, contemplating the rock formations. The small grey stones were finely raked into swirling parallel rows, with strategically placed ornate rocks creating the effect of an ocean scene. James didn't know how long he had been out there, when he was woken from his revelry by the muted sound of a car starting, engaging its gears and driving off. He couldn't believe it when he looked out on the driveway and Maria's car was gone. A small note on the living room table said: 'I need some space. I'll be in Saratoga if you want to reach me'.

Maria's parents were overjoyed at the return of their daughter. They were thinking that maybe things were finally turning out the way they planned and their patience was at last rewarded. Maria had never hated her parents, just accepted that they all had a different point of view. Her father's stubborn resistance to accept James after his daughter had lived with this man was a front for the anger toward James's chosen profession and the industry's practices. Or maybe Luigi resented that James had amassed a fortune as great as or greater than his, in a relatively fast time and was driving him from his land in the process.

Maria maintained an uneasy truce with her parents by not mentioning James's name around the house. While her return was a cause for family celebration, it didn't take too long for Roberto to come over from the beach and make use of the change in dynamics. He had been lobbying for some action and now that there was an opening, he cornered Maria's father after lunch at the golf club. "You won't have a business to manage soon because all your trees will be gone. If you don't make a stand now, there will be no orchards left in this valley."

"We already made our petition to the governor after the last demonstration and he is reviewing it. He says he's big on the environment so let's see what he says. I don't think another action will help at this point," Luigi said reaching for his wine.

"You know how it is in Sacramento. Governor Brown

is introducing all these new programs and needs the new technology folks behind him. He may talk like an environmentalist but we both know what backroom deals get made in the name of progress. I say you need to show him the problem here is real." Roberto tossed his napkin on the table like he was drawing a line he dared Luigi to cross.

"Maybe you have a point there," Luigi said rising to the bait.

"If we don't stand together, we'll be walked on again. If you let this kid get away with it, everyone else in the valley will think they can do the same," Roberto said with a hint of passion not wanting to oversell his plan.

"Maybe you're right—"

"Of course I am. Now listen." Roberto leaned in confidentially. "This Eden Computers is planning to go on the stock exchange. I think if we can initiate some negative publicity, the offering will get pulled and the punk can go back to fixing toasters in his garage." He looked at Luigi evenly like his suggestion had merit.

Luigi was reluctant but now that his daughter didn't seem to be involved anymore he didn't have to risk offending her. Roberto leveraged Maria's return as the impetus, suggesting starting an attack before she changed her mind and went back to the other camp.

15

THE CHRISTMAS CHILD

El Niño was making its semi-annual Christmas visit to Los Angeles with a ferocity that left quick-tongued weathermen stumbling over their words, as this petulant child from below the equator cried gallons of water a second on the Southland. It was Noah's Ark weather, a tropical storm that flung itself unabated at the California coast, with endless days and nights of rain falling in heavy, miserable waves. The traffic crawling on the freeways inched along slower than ever, wading through flooded roadways. Rivers of muddy water transformed staid communities of orderly and conservative houses into Third World hurricane ghettos.

From Beverly Hills to Pacific Palisades and from Laguna Beach to Santa Barbara, the rich and famous mansions were as deluged as the lowliest homes in the flatlands of the LA basin. Everybody living on a slope had to sandbag their homes against encroaching water. Flights at LAX were disrupted and the Coast Highway was flooded in places. And where the steep hills met the ocean, mudslides blocked sections of the road, while exposing boulders the size of small houses that threatened to tumble from eroded cliffs onto the reluctant traffic.

On a tree-covered ridge above Malibu Canyon, a contemporary styled house overlooking its classy neighbors down on the beach was being secured against the attack of El Niño. The house belonged to a wealthy rock star named Vance Champlain, and directing the handyman who was putting plastic storm sheeting on the windows was Vance's newest tenant, Roscoe Malone.

Vance had permanently relocated to Maui a year before and was renting his house to Malone and his newlywed wife, Hart Akers. Hart knew Vance from the record company where she worked and he gave her a friendly deal. He didn't really need the money because of all the royalties from a couple of Top Ten songs written during his time in a sixties pop group whose songs were recognizable standards like many other one-hit wonders. He had been looking for someone responsible who would act more like a house sitter, so rented it out for next to nothing. Hart had been dating Roscoe in a whirlwind romance that developed in parallel to Stephan's developing relationship with Lila only ending up with opposite results. Malone didn't miss a beat when the house came up for rent suggesting he and Hart share the rent and a new level of opportunities presented themselves.

Stephan was up to his neck in hot mineral water at the Tradewinds Spa in Desert Hot Springs, explaining all this to Sid, the young and playful spa manager. Soaking next to him was her perpetual suitor Harry Hogarth, the band's coke dealer on one of his endless quests to get Sid in bed. Stephan was in the desert for a couple of weeks to work on keeping the publishing business alive now that it had been moved there after the storms took away the Malibu house where it and the other businesses had been relocated. The storm's damage had forced Malone into permanent residency at his vacation home in the desert. Stephan went on to explain to Sid how Malone had landed one of the most desirable babes in LA – the Jiva band's original Artists & Repertoire representative.

"You think Malone saw Hart in his future when he calculated his horoscope?" Harry asked.

"I wouldn't give him that much credit," Sid said. "But when it comes to the green stuff and living well off others, he certainly has a nose for it."

"I guess his emerald really is lucky. Look who he ended up with," Stephan said.

Hart was a natural blond Valley Girl with a tall, thin physique and full bust line that many compared to a Barbie doll figure. Hart was the privileged daughter of a successful set of parents whose commercial real-estate empire ranged from modern office parks in Orange County to extensive industrial sites by Long Beach. The family estate was on the valley side of LA, tucked into a small canyon in Encino. Hart's parents divorced when she was in her late teens so hers was a lonely upbringing. She lost herself in music and eventually got a degree in it at UCLA's music industry program. Hart was ambitious and smart, which combined with her good looks, landed her a job at A&M Records as an executive secretary which then led to a role as an Artist Relations manager. Hart wasn't intimidated by fame or fortune and could deal with big-name rock stars as well as the executives running the company, retaining enough respect to not appear arrogant. She was able to be frank and yet at the same time caring and attentive. Initially hired to be eye candy she ended up impressing her bosses (Mr. Alpert and Mr. Moss) with her intelligence. They also learned to respect Hart as her intuitive decisions for new creative directions kept the sensitive artists happy.

Hart's first assignment as an A&R person was to baby-sit a promising band brought to the label by one of their megastars, George Harrison. She worked alongside the producer and engineer and kept track of the making of the record. After the recording was completed, Hart animated the sales and radio promotion departments, getting them excited about the album so the band just might have a hit. Hart preferred to be close to the action and the chance to be part of something big made her coddle Jiva and get them through their first record and related activities without too much trauma. And then one fateful night at a party north of Sunset, deep in Coldwater Canyon that was packed with musicians, music executives, groupies and starlets, she connected with Roscoe Malone. He was suave, stylish and good with his words and manners but also a hero in her eyes after a comic or heroic rescue, depending on where you were standing. He had average looks but personality made up for appearances in a town short on substance and long on image.

"Everyone was loaded, so the show looked cool and nobody was in a state to judge Malone's athletic prowess," Harry said.

"But he did save the guy's life," Sid said reaching for

her iced tea.

"No question," Harry said. "The producer fell in the pool and he was such a clown everyone thought he was joking with all his splashing around but he was actually drowning." He made some exaggerated arm movements to illustrate the scene.

"Then Malone waded in the shallow end and managed to reach the guy and pull him out." Stephan went on to explain how Malone had been attracted to Hart after seeing her handle the band at a couple of showcases, so they were already acquaintances. When she congratulated him on his rescue and brought him a snifter of brandy to fight off a chill, the stage was set.

"There sure were a long line of admirers in addition to Malone," Harry said.

"And were you one of them?" Sid asked. Her question hid the occasional insecurity she felt about her tomboy figure and average looks when compared to the Hollywood girls who passed through the spa.

"Naw, not me. She was like a sister," Harry said with innocent eyes to an unconvinced looking Sid as he reached for his beer.

"I have to admit I wasn't immune to her charms either but I was already dating Lila," Stephan said while pushing himself out of the water to sit on the edge of the pool.

Malone had started to date Hart after their encounter at the party. While he found her attractive and charming his instinct for homing in on individuals with wealth and privilege meant her family tree hadn't gone unnoticed. Then in a spontaneous moment when the two of them bumped into each other in a Hollywood drugstore, their low-key mutual attraction sparked and led them to fly to Vegas for a quick marriage.

Their new home in Malibu was a modern split-level ranch house with a redwood and tile interior, hidden amongst stands of eucalyptus trees and dense vegetation. It was situated on the side of a steep canyon ridge, facing southwest to catch the sunsets over the neighbors' mansions and taking in a smoggy vista of Palos Verdes peninsula to the south or on exceptional days, Catalina Island.

Hart stepped back from the wild life of trying to keep up with bands whose sole occupation when not on stage was partying away their money and spent more time in the office than on the road. A sense of domesticity slowly took hold, with the occasional wild party usually hosted as a fundraiser for social causes. The most recent event had gotten the police to show up as Tom Petty and the Heartbreakers rocked so loud the neighbors across the canyon were complaining.

With the oil embargo from mad Arabs creating long lines at gas stations across the country still a memory and a possible repeat threat, Malone decided to move the calendar productions up to the house to save on his commuting. A drawing table was installed in the large bay window section of the guest bedroom that Vance called the meditation room. Stephan spent many late nights fueled by the house blend Kona coffee, putting together a marketing plan and composing mails to promote the ultimate guide to human existence from an astrological perspective. Some nights he would camp out in 'the pit', a sunken living room full of cushions, decorated like a pasha's salon. The future was bright until the clouds that drifted in as part of the weather pattern triggered by warm ocean currents from South America, started dumping tons of water without end.

El Niño's tantrum raged on full throttle, and up at the top of Malibu Canyon, Malone played captain of the ship, battening down the hatches of Vance's spread, to weather out the deluge. A couple of big groups of eucalyptus provided a natural barrier and the house also had a low, angular profile allowing it to avoid getting too beat up by the wind. The windows still rattled and when the wind blasted in from over the ocean driving the rain sideways, trickles of water seeped in around the window frames where the glass buckled and warped under the pressure of the high winds. Another millimeter of pressure and the glass would have shattered like being hit by a large hammer. The newlyweds hunkered down in 'the pit' where the small windows and low profile from being partially buried in the hillside made it a sort of bunker.

Malone had Jerry, their outdoorsman handyman, ferry up supplies in one of the International Harvester 4x4s while the storm raged. Every day Jerry removed fallen tree branches from the private road. After the first week of non-stop rain, he routinely shoveled away the silt and gravel that washed down the hillside and was continually building up in a pile against the inside of the electric gate. By then LA County had been declared a federal disaster area and finally the power lines went down, forcing

Malone and Hart to abandon ship and set up a temporary base in a hotel over in the San Fernando Valley.

Stephan had been busy in the office doing production activities and running around to meetings at the TV station for their in-house newsletter so was immune to a possible work blockage due to inaccessibility to the workroom in Malibu. Getting to Hollywood from the Westside took time but his trusty Honda plowed through the water like a speedboat. He had to put in a lot of hours, as it was late in the season for shipping *Star Sign* calendars and the last-minute orders had to be assembled for waiting customers.

Stephan received the disaster call when it became clear the hillside Vance's house was built on was rapidly eroding into a river of brown earth. The fill dirt underneath half of the main building had become so saturated after ten days of soaking that it liquefied and followed the force of gravity to the bottom of the canyon. The foundation of the house shifted and as if a large pair of hands was tearing it in half, and the house cracked down the middle from the roof through to the floor. One half shifted with the moving earth, twisting to a tilted angle with the rooms' contents crashing through the windows and the redwood strips in the ceiling splintering and snapping with loud cracks like gunshots.

Stephan helped the resourceful Jerry salvage as much as could be safely recovered, like Vance's old photos from band tours, his guitar collection and stage clothing. By the third day the house was too dangerous to go into. The county had condemned the building days earlier but that hadn't deterred them from carrying on with their duties. Now the operation was over and after the storm subsided, bulldozers were called in to level the remaining parts of the house to discourage any scavengers or curiosity seekers from entering the ruined structure.

Vance had never spent more than a couple of weeks a year there, preferring his Hawaiian hacienda, so there was no sentimental attachment. It was fully insured, so no need to cry over the loss. He had bought the place from some hotshot lawyer for only one point five million, so easy come, easy go.

Malone took the hit harder, having made the place into his own residence and had started to identify with it as an extension of his successful image. During those two weeks a year when Vance was in town they had camped out in hotels or else stayed in the weekend house in the desert. Now the fallback plan was re-establishing Malone's emerging kingdom in the wide-open spaces an hour and a half west of Los Angeles. Like a lot of Angelinos looking to escape the late spring and early summer coastal fog, the area by Palm Springs had become a standard retreat with its 364 days of sun a year.

Malone had set his sights for empire building on Desert Hot Springs, a small resort community about fifteen miles from Palm Springs, built into the low foothills of the Joshua Tree Monument's western boundary. The fault lines zigzagging the state had blessed this region with hot mineral water just below the surface that found its way up through the various fissures. Tourism was the main industry, with a variety of spa-tels – hotels that were health spas – if chlorine-enhanced mineral water could be considered curative.

Malone's vision of an empire would lead him to become the mayor of this sleepy backwater. His beachhead was taking over the top floor of a worn-out looking two-story building on the main street. Home base was a modest suburban ranch house on the edge of the desert, where the developments ended in tumbleweeds and sagebrush. Malone wanted to visibly build up his businesses to establish his credibility. This would put him on his way to becoming a civic leader in a town he believed was poised to become a major tourist area, with the right promotion and local government leadership. He had a vision of golf courses and a healthy image of sun and mineral water cures creating a clean industry as a base for further expansion.

The trouble was that the cash cow funding the growth of Malone's corporate infrastructure had gone to pasture, in fact more like to the slaughterhouse. Malone had been successfully courting investors for his oil schemes to fund corporate expansion. Part of the ritual was high-profile dinners at the Malibu house, with whatever well-known musician they could find in attendance to give an air of glamour to the event. It also helped show Malone had connections and the house itself was impressive enough to wow most people and make them think they too could enjoy similar perks if they invested as the apparently wise Malone had. Never mind the artists were contacts of Hart's and the house belonged to her friend, Malone carried on without Hart suspecting that the dinner parties had a second purpose rather than just socializing. The earlier oil crisis created interest in fuel sources closer to home, so Malone's ownership certificates in Mexican oil futures seemed like savvy investments to cash-rich customers looking to hedge their money.

It was all about image and winning through intimidation, so with a sharp suit and spectacular home, the appearance of success was obvious. Now without a base of operations to lure new unsuspecting patrons, the funding dried up to pay the original oil subscribers' dividends. Malone turned to the next deep-pocketed sponsor waiting to be helped with spending their abundant amounts of cash – the federal government.

With LA County declared a national disaster area, homeowners and businesspeople impacted by the storm were eligible to receive loans with a minimal interest of around one percent, in essence – free money. Malone hit the Feds with his own El Niño downpour of loan applications for all his many businesses and he also filled one out for him and his wife, encouraging Stephan to do the same. After all, the design facilities had been relocated to Vance's during the oil crisis and Stephan had spent enough nights there to qualify as a resident.

Stephan hadn't seen the forms that Malone had filled out, and it was only when Malone presented the application for Great Impressions at a meeting in the office that Stephan got an idea about what was going on. The inventory list showed a lot more than a beat-up drawing table purloined from the studio. There was binding equipment, IBM Selectric typewriters, printed publications valued at near retail costs, art supplies, research books, original designs and so many other incidentals. An extra two pages were attached to list everything.

"We can't submit this, it's a bunch of bullshit," Stephan said challenging the stack of papers.

"I'll admit that there is some padding here and there, but you have to see we're in this unique moment in time where the cards we've been dealt give us a chance to go for a winning hand. The money will give us the chance to finally get this company off the ground, the way it should be set up. We could never get this much cash out of a bank." Malone was sitting behind his large desk projecting success, dressed in polo shirt and slacks, as was the more customary formal attire in the desert.

"I know we need to build up our operation, but this is like forgery. We're faking information and if we get caught it's a federal offense. If this gets investigated we won't just get our loan tuned down like at a bank – we'll get some hard time in a penitentiary because this is the US government here." Stephan shifted to the edge of the office chair preparing to leave.

"Look, I had the same thought but there's no way they will ever find out what was or wasn't in the house. It's gone – totaled – history. And nobody is going digging. If it will make you happy, just remember this is in fact a loan and we will pay it back with the requested interest. You know we both pay enough taxes. Us ordinary citizens should finally get a break and have a temporary share of what's out there. Imagine the ads we can buy, the designers we can hire, as well as the talent we can attract." Malone gestured expansively as if waving away the image of the beat-up office with a more modern version replacing it.

"I just don't like lying, that's all. When I was in India my teacher said: 'When you speak, always speak the truth and when you write, always write the truth'."

"Wise man, I like that. Okay, I'll go along with your honesty trip. You're always saying this is all an illusion and not to take it seriously, so why are you ignoring your own advice?"

"You're joking, right?" Stephan looked at Malone like he was crazy. "This is attached to a huge lie. I can't accept this." Stephan stood up and thrust his hands in his jeans pockets.

"You want to stay a starving artist and see the business you invested so much time in fall by the wayside when we can get temporary use of some cash, all for embellishing a story? Hell, you're a writer fur crissake. You're writing fiction, so get off your moral high horse and be practical for once. We can even get a professional editor for your story and a decent marketing budget. Send you on a twenty-city book tour. Or would you rather have your masterpiece end up forgotten? We're not stealing and if we were, don't you think Uncle Sam could afford it?"

Stephan sighed deeply but maintained his resistance. "I'm still not convinced – the potential for trouble is bigger than any eventual reward." Malone was angry and got up and stormed off past Stephan and eventually filed the papers for the business including Great Impressions without Stephan's participation. It took weeks for Malone to talk to Stephan civilly because he was sure the government would have given them more money if Stephan had also participated. He was apparently counting on getting a share of Stephan's personal loan, if he had applied for one.

Bingo – in no time at all there were hundreds of thousands of dollars in taxpayer's money to fund the expansion of the desert empire. The federal government had stepped in at a convenient time. Malone was already contemplating a run on a bank (having burned through all his credit cards) for financing Globall Corporation, the parent company that owned all the various small businesses. This would have involved fake inventory papers and sales figures, but the disaster loans were less demanding in required documentation. With the huge number of applications, the federal loan agency couldn't get into too much detail and check each request. With the Malibu home bulldozed, Malone was a clear disaster victim, and who was going to dig through the rubble to verify all the lost calendar production equipment that never existed and shoe inventory that still remained at the studio.

Born to the task of spending money as though he had a printing press in the basement cranking out Franklins, Malone hired an editor and designer. And now with the funding to seriously build a business, the plans for expanding the line of published materials and ability to market and fund projects suddenly made Stephan's months of sweat and toil look like they were finally being rewarded. No more day jobs, just focusing on the business of building the company that was already showing signs of success. Stephan was commuting but spending weeks at a time in a doublewide trailer Malone was renting for the revolving staff members. Whenever Hart was on one of her frequent visits to LA to keep an eye on the couple of bands she was mothering, Stephan and Malone would cruise in a four-wheel drive through desert arroyos. Malone would spout shaman wisdom as if he had studied with Carlos Castaneda's mystical teacher from Mexico, Don Juan.

The *Star Sign Calendar* had reached forty-seven of the fifty states and they had talked about international distribution after a few sales in England. And as their mainstay was a calendar, there was talk about branching out into executive organizers with removable sections that a businessperson could customize to their needs. Naturally an executive 'tool' would also include the moneymaking wisdom from the mind of the financial genius Roscoe Malone. To top off the good news, a large major publisher Stephan had initiated discussions with about the possibility of licensing the calendar as a franchise, was sounding very serious. This would mean not only funding, but also nationwide distribution with support from the publisher's sales reps.

Their local evening hangout was a spa-tel named the Tradewinds that had been taken over by a gay hairdresser from Hollywood when his aunt left it to him in her will. It was a classic spa on the edge of the desert with a large square indoor hot tub of pure mineral water and an outdoor pool that was the oasis for the sun worshippers. The new owner had it managed by Sid, with a reputation of an outrageous party girl who had bounced between the west coast hot spots and Hawaii. She soon had it packed on the weekends with film crews on break and every type of high-life creature who wanted a change of scene from the burn-out life in Tinseltown.

The parties would start Friday night and wind down Sunday afternoon when the exodus to LA started again. Stephan had spent many wild weekends there before the offices had relocated, so knew the crew well. One of Sid's friends was an aspiring actress who had starred in *Video Girls*, a two-hour music video posing as a movie and she had taken a liking to Stephan that made frequent visits easy. They never consummated their mutual attraction as Stephan was in his goddess worshipping mode, reluctant to seek anything serious after his frustrating times with Lila, another actress.

It was better during the week when the indoor tub wasn't full of drunks and the locals could have space to kick back. Occasionally some drug smuggling desert rats would visit, keeping very much to themselves. They were people Sid knew from a past life living on a small island off the coast. Their desert camouflage off-road vehicles would rumble by in the dead of night after a rendezvous with a small plane that either landed on a dry lakebed or simply tossed out bales of marijuana on a low-level pass.

Malone and Stephan would typically start the day with a jog in the desert to get energized. They were living the dream others could only imagine possible of residing in a resort environment and catching the opportunities it presented in the early stage of development, building a set of businesses as the bedrock for becoming solid citizens.

Stephan was slowly drawn into using his editing skills to support the other schemes of Globall. He found himself spending less time on his writing and felt guilty as he was drifting from his original goal of sharing the wisdom from the silent baba.

Malone targeted the money they had received from the government at expansion on all fronts, so the publishing money soon disappeared into a common pot. A professionally designed front cover for the new *Star Sign Calendar* was one item that benefited from the cash infusion. Earlier versions were handmade creations where antique reproductions were cut out of an art book and glued on a page. Now a real designer under the guidance of a producer, who managed ad designs for his own agency, was putting together something commercial and slick looking, in full color.

All systems were 'go' and the pieces were in place to become financially independent, with a variety of enterprises poised for imminent growth. There was just one small issue that cropped up with the potential to spoil the party – Uncle Sam knocking on the door asking for repayment of the loans.

Stephan made the occasional trip back to the big city for a reality check and to see if either of his songs was going to be put out as a single. He had sub-let his bungalow for a couple of months so when he visited the Gardens he slept on Maceo's sofa – a guest in his own neighborhood. On his latest trek to Blem Gardens Stephan wandered over to Reedo and Jack's bungalow one evening as the low heat and cramped quarters had made it impossible to stay indoors. He found the two residents engaged in a feverish game of backgammon, fueled by nacho-flavored Doritos and Danish beer. They broke off the game and invited Stephan in and told him about last month's major events in the life of a rock and roll band.

Of course they started talking about Hart who had been looking after them in typical outfits like tight jeans and translucent silk blouses that drove Reedo crazy. Her calm presence kept the rest of the band on their best gentlemanly behavior whenever she was around. Taking care of their needs from the very beginning, she had worked with Jiva at the Record Plant, the pre-eminent studio of choice for everyone from successful seventies stadium bands to British invasion dregs.

The recording had gone well with the usual hobnobbing with neighboring acts like the Eagles or Stevie Wonder sharing the jacuzzis and party rooms. Jack and Reedo never knew who they would bump into in the hallway. One day it was an angel-haired balladeer from an art band, and the next, a leather-and-chain-wearing heavy metal thrasher. The band held their own, and jammed with their heroes, sharing war stories of life on the road, and record-label gripes. The Record Plant was the center of LA rock and roll music recording, with every accommodation made to support the artistic process. Reedo explained that the band liked hanging out in the billiards room that was complete with an old soda machine, dispensing beers for ten cents. The additional price of admission was that they also had to put up with the mad antics of Keith Moon and his guitar crashing lead guitarist from the legendary British band, The Who.

Jiva finally got the album finished, with some help from a couple of session players. The production was polished and it still retained a spark of their live energy. The band was taken out to a dry lakebed in the Mojave Desert where a lot of album covers and commercials got shot. They posed their way through a photo session, to create their version of an album cover. The group peered petulantly into the camera's eye with their bare torsos and windblown hair highlighted by the pinkish hues from a desert sunset that colored the lunar landscape. Jack proudly told how he convinced everyone afterwards to visit his desert hideaway for a huge barbeque.

Airplay was positive following the initial release of the album, and their signature song 'Something's Goin' On Inside, LA' was climbing towards the Top Ten in only two weeks. The band had been checking *Billboard* magazine every week, hoping that sales would build and that they could each get fat royalty checks for a hit single. Jack soon realized that to build a following, they needed to get on the road. Negotiating with Alan and George, they were able to get a slot as the opening act for Fleetwood Mac, a British blues band whose leader was a former boyfriend of George's sister. The headlining band's tour had been momentarily upset when their opening act took off to do their own solo tour. Jiva was quickly accepted as a replacement, and soon scheduled to set off for Atlanta to join Mac on the road.

The allure of a band that had some buzz attached to it attracted all types of people, eager to be a part of the story, including those who provided party materials. One character that everyone knew as The Count slowly became integrated into the scene at Jiva's local shows. Harry Hogarth was tall, with a Germanic air of cool sophistication but was actually from Chicago. He wasn't any type of royalty, the adopted name simply referred to his tendency to never get the count right, always providing a little less than the agreed amount of product in a deal. Nobody made a fuss, as he had shared so many lines of coke with the groupies and fans that it was ridiculous to haggle over some crumbs.

The Count would periodically drop by Blem after he finished school for the day at the gemological institute he was studying at. If nobody else was around, he would check in on Stephan, and share a beer or else try and convince him to join in for a cruise of some new punk music bars that evening. The rough and tumble clubs were opening up on Main Street in Santa Monica, in the run-down strip of real estate of the polarized Ocean Park district, trying to be a beachside Brentwood rather than a crime-ridden Venice. The Count liked Stephan's company, and he didn't have to disappear so often in the men's room to pack his nose, because there was minimal interest from Stephan in Peruvian alkaloids. That meant Harry could chill for a change and spare his nervous system a few extra jolts. Stephan always shared inspiring words from his research that had the potential to shift the focus to inner contentment. And when the nights got too quiet and

Stephan started to think about calling Lila, Harry would take him down to Main Street. There they would visit a few bars to distract themselves and Stephan was entertained by watching Harry endlessly chatting up women. He liked the way Harry was fearless and open in his flirting and over time Stephan had some short-lived adventures with a few ladies on the periphery of the scene. There was an artist who was more interested in sex than painting and the bartender in Redondo Beach who seduced him with a pitcher of margaritas while watching TV on her king-sized bed. The encounters had been fun but he avoided any commitment as he was still holding out for the one true love. And this usually meant thinking about where Lila might be.

Stephan felt himself drifting, not sure what version of reality to call home. The desert offered some signs of hope and he had planned to use the solitude to reconnect to his writing but felt blocked. Like James, getting deep into the business world meant his pure focus on writing some enlightening story was being diluted, especially when he felt exhausted from his day job. He missed the closeness with Lila and their talks where she acted as his muse, making the writing work seem more urgent and real. By contrast, Malone looked at Stephan's story as a hobby and wasn't particularly supportive. Even being back in Blem wasn't really inspiring him with creative motivation as the band kept disappearing on tour and Maceo was in a phase of endless research.

When the inspiration fired him up and he was working on the Rama story, rereading sections of the epic brought back memories of his trip to India and in particular the test by fire. The nightmare vision of someone dying before his eyes was as vivid in his imagination as the day he witnessed it. He tried to comprehend the finality of death and the end of an individual's existence. That image in turn would take him back to the race and seeing the crumpled body of Tobias. He had only slightly more connection with the dead racer than the Indian girl but it troubled him more as it had become personal due to his friend's involvement. Unlike Greg, Stephan had created a new existence in LA that had replaced his earlier life in the Bay Area. Home became a relative concept and his current location of the moment his only reality. He knew he could create his story anywhere with the right spark to kick him onwards but was using the excuse of all his issues to wallow in the exquisite feeling of writer's block, while in the waiting room for Doctor Inspiration.

16

THE BABY BLUE FLAKE COSMIC COLORED STREAMLINED BABY

Santa Cruz was a town that still had the vestiges of a Wild West mythos, where lumberjacks and deep-sea fishermen shared the sidewalks with surfers, wide-eyed university students and the hard-working John Q. Citizens, dodging panhandling hippies who still thought it was 1967. Stephan's infrequent visits to the seaside resort town bordered by ancient redwoods and a wild rocky coastline were on one hand refreshing after the LA sprawl and yet disorienting as a walk in the low laying fog. The place was suspended in a time warp where not much ever seemed to change, making any reference point useless.

Visiting James on Stephan's trips north had become less and less of an option, as James had gotten so far into his business that other than a quick coffee (or in James's case a Miso soup) there wasn't much time for any meaningful contact. As a result, Stephan had also lost track of Maria, as he usually saw her when he would visit James on a lazy Sunday afternoon. Now with the Eden business growing and competitors revving up their product lines, there was no day of rest. Stephan had enjoyed the easy conversation and even though they didn't talk about India too much, he liked hearing about James's new fascination with Japanese-flavored Buddhism.

Stephan guessed that one motivation for James's interest was partly to discover the Eastern way of thinking that allowed Japanese companies like Sony to tap into universal human needs and combine the best of existing technology elements and create popular consumer devices like tiny transistor radios and Trinitron color televisions.

When Stephan met James and Maria on those earlier occasions, the talks were always inspired and would vary from the Zen goal of mindfulness of the present moment to the fool's journey in the land of Maria's pentacles and spades that represented the development of human potential. Stephan would share his latest research from the world of yoga philosophy, echoing the oneness of all things. Stephan regretfully gave up trying to reach James after half a dozen calls and knew a visit to the offices would mean a less than fifty percent chance of finding James, as he was always in outside meetings these days. On this visit, he went straight over to Santa Cruz when he landed to find Greg.

It was a chilly foggy day by the beach as Stephan banged a few times on the weathered front door of Greg's run-down house, with its neglected lawn and dried-up hedges. He jammed his hands into his jeans pockets to keep warm, while he waited as the sun tried to find its way through the high fog. A Dodge Dart and an Impala were rusting in the driveway alongside the house, both with gaping holes where their engines and hood covers had been removed.

The door opened reluctantly and Greasy greeted Stephan bleary-eyed with a hearty, "Hey, spud nose!" and gave him a big hug. "Let's start the party. We were waiting for our honored guest to arrive to get this place rocking. C'mon in, put your feet up, relax and enjoy the view. Got a big event tonight – a birthday party for two crazy brothers from New Jersey with a Dolly Parton look-alike live and in person. Maybe it's even really Dolly. What is reality will be the Zen question of the evening. After enough beers you'll believe anything, I guarantee it. I tell ya, reality is relative."

"Oh, yeah? I think relativity is real." Stephan sat on a shabby sofa and watched Greg pacing the room in his baggy jeans, white T-shirt and an unbuttoned plaid Pendleton wool shirt, flapping like wings behind him.

"Well yes, I would hope so, big city boy, student of the scriptures and seducer of stars. Remember Emery? Come here, pretty kitty." Greg motioned for his petite girlfriend with ratty hair to join them, when he saw her passing in the hallway in a worn-out faded blue bathrobe. She waved him away and carried on in a sleepy shuffle.

"C'mon and spread those yams, mama!" Greg called after her and then turning to Stephan said, "Being a vegetarian I can't say spread those hams, gotta be yams. And when she's shy about swallowing after a blowjob, I have to tell her 'don't panic, it's organic'. We just got up so why don't we go make us some breakfast."

It was four in the afternoon.

By six they were in the first of what would be a series of run-down neighborhood bars that hadn't bothered to invest in updating their furniture or décor as the locals didn't mind. Greg introduced Stephan to all the counterculture's finest who were already too wasted to be conversational or overtly outrageous in their hyper-articulated phrasing due to being drunk. Greg would massage the egos, guide the prima donnas to a point where they were tolerated by the masses and even get the most withdrawn pothead to contribute a few words. Greg did this in a whirlwind of conversation and antics using every available prop to add to the performance. Greg was echoing the Pranksters' philosophy of finding the cool place in each person and helping let it shine. Through the blur of alcohol and grass Stephan was too disoriented to see if this evening was a special event just for him or Greg's usual lifestyle. If this was the standard routine Stephan was sure that it was a downward spiral, a glossed-over nosedive into oblivion where the altimeter was spinning wildly measuring the descent.

The problems had started for Greg when he needed to slow down his jangling nerves from driving all day and night buzzed on crank, so a little H became the antidote. Without any better guidance from his circle of friends, and Stephan's lack of understanding of the seriousness of the dependency that had developed, Greg's slide deeper into opiate dreamland had carried on. Greasy joked, jived, slapped backs and gave people special names in his continuing one-man circus, so it was hard to tell where the limits were. But as usual, Greasy the inner explorer wanted to push the edge, see where the limits really ended and move beyond.

On his last visit north when Stephan had caught up with Greg, they were in his living room swapping stories and it had become clear to Stephan that Greg was strung out. Greg could maintain his composure as if everything was normal but to someone from outside the scene it was more than obvious. In a mix of anger and compassion Stephan had finally lost his restraint after all the small talk and launched into Greg.

"Man, what the fuck is going on? You look like you're trying to swim underwater with weights on and your brain is running in reverse. If you think you're being cool it ain't so."

Greg replied staring ahead out the window as if they were talking about someone else, "I really do 'preciate your concern but you're blowing things up way out of proportion. I hear you but I'm no junkie – I can walk away at any time. It's just a little medicine to take the edge off, if you know what I mean."

"Last time I was here you were much more alive and now you look like a zombie." Stephan turned his body for emphasis looking directly at Greg.

"I'm telling ya, don't exaggerate the situation. Yeah, I do give myself a muscle jab here and there but it's not mainlining. And whenever I walk away from the shit it's the same as having the flu for a couple of days. That's it." Greg replied with a shrug looking at Stephan like they were talking about the weather.

"I don't care if you have the shits for a week when you quit, you're slowly destroying yourself. And I don't mean just your body. I'm no pharmacologist but you're also doing your head in. And if you think we're ever going to be good yogis and start a center for helping people you really are strung out. Nobody's going to come within a million miles of you in this state – you reek of junkie. Sure, you're groovy and cool with all the locals but that's a show. When you're giving everyone your cosmic universal love and brotherhood rap 'cause you're feeling mellow what you don't see an hour later is everyone saying to each other about what a strung-out, burnt-out loser you are. Talking a holy talk and knowing some Indian philosophy doesn't qualify you to be above the masses. Not if you are jabbing yourself with a needle every day."

Greg had stopped looking at Stephan and hung his head taking it in. Stephan went on in a gentler tone about shifting the focus and remembering the sanctity of the body as the house for the God energy each human had a spark of inside. After Stephan had made his point they had made their peace but how deep Stephan's words had gone wasn't sure.

Stephan's other main show of support was to take Greg to the Staff of Life health food store, and buy a couple of bags of wholesome foods to stock Greg's kitchen with in hopes of giving him a decent diet to support a cure. Brown rice and miso to remove toxins with tofu and brewer's yeast for protein and organic bread and vegetables rounded out the menu. Stephan would clean the kitchen with the stereo blasting and prepare a pile of food, feeling hopeful when he saw Greg energized after a solid meal, when a spark of Greg's old self would shine through.

After making the rounds at the local bars they sat around

the kitchen table waiting to see who would drop by. The house was always hosting a rotating cast of characters attracted to Greg's open lifestyle. People liked hearing his folksy wisdom in late night rap sessions.

Stephan had finished an update on the band's latest adventures, as Greg was always interested in their progress. Emery rolled a joint and wandered off to the living room to play solitaire while watching some TV. Greg got up and made a show of investigating the cabinets like he was going to prepare some food. He found a bag of Oreos and popped one in his mouth before holding out the bag to Stephan.

"Thanks, but it's a little early in the day for me." Stephan knew a craving for sugar was a sign of heroin use.

"Just imagine they're buckwheat with a tofu filling," Greg said before munching another one and putting the bag away.

"If they were, you could make a killing selling them to James." They both laughed. "You never used to be a sweet freak. Is this some kind of medical ailment?"

"Just a measure of pure pleasure. Chocolate and cream, to help me dream."

"As long as your dreams tonight are cookies and not poppies I'll be happy."

"Dude, the flower ain't got power at this hour so don't look so sour."

Stephan was happy to see that the other periodic residents of Greg's house, Jim and Carla, were absent. They were Santa Cruz locals, as far back as several generations. It took about three visits before they stopped considering

Stephan a 'Val' from the valley over the hill and for Stephan to figure out Carla wasn't a secretary but actually a stripper in a topless bar by the pier. It meant she was probably also selling her body for the right amount of money.

The living room was bare compared to Stephan's last visit, when evidence of the crew's latest nocturnal adventures was scattered around. That time it was crumpled beer cans and an empty nitrous oxide tank leaning against the wall that was stolen the night before from a dentist's office. The misfits had gone there in search of any kind of medication, hopeful to find some downers like Percodan or Diladin. Jim had taken Stephan aside and valiantly defended his role as a friend who was helping clean up Greg. He and Carla had been the main benefactors of Greg's largesse, but slowly the income had been dropping which translated into their being around less and less.

Stephan asked Greg why the house seemed so empty and there were fewer cars in the driveway than usual.

"Gotta blame my boss. Thought Bernie was my friend but claims my driving ain't up to scratch – so not doing as many runs as usual."

"At least you're able to pay the rent."

"That's not a problem. When times got tough I sold this dump to a buddy who invests in real estate and I'm the official caretaker in exchange for paying rent. I make the odd dollar selling some stuff—"

"Stuff?" Stephan said cutting him off.

"You know, a little this, a little that."

"Looks to me like you're dipping into the product a bit."

"One of the benefits, I say. Helping yourself while

helping others."

"But where did that monster set of speakers go?"

"Same place as my baby-blue Porsche – my local supporters."

"The one with the cosmic-colored blue flake paint job we did all those cruises in?"

"Don't you worry – she's still around when we want to take a spin."

They went back in the kitchen after looking in on Emery who was engrossed with her card game, deftly sidestepping an overflowing cat box in the midst of piles of empty beer and vodka bottles.

"How 'bout some spuds then? They're cheap and you can fix them a hundred ways. Got to save the cash for stash, if you know what I mean."

"I know. Times are tough all over."

"Spuds, spuds, spuds, spuds…" Greg sang in a low octave like an army song, while he marched a fifty-pound sack of potatoes out of the pantry.

Stephan looked in the near empty refrigerator that's sole contents were a variety of condiments.

Greg said, "Time to go shopping. Don't worry; we'll be eating in a flash. So tell me, when can I read your book? I want to see if it turns out the same way as the original, with the Rama guy getting his girl back untouched by the ten-headed dude. It's so righteous you're writing that. A lesson in love in a loveless world."

"It's taking longer than I thought, but step by step I'll finish it."

"Cool. And still twisting the ol' body into knots like a

good sadhu?" Greg said.

"Trying. I go to this teacher named Bilkem, who has a fast-moving style of yoga he calls ShaktiFlow©®™."

"Sounds very Lost Angeles. I got something I call go-slow yoga." He laughed at his private joke. "Hey, I didn't tell you, I've lined you up a little muse to inspire you. A cute babe that will melt your heart. We'll go meet her after we're done eating. You can practice your hatha yoga and try some yogi foreplay: 'hey baby, cross your legs behind your head and smile'." Greg was looking through a countertop piled with dirty dishes and glasses, locating the potato peeler that he rinsed, started in on a pile of potatoes.

"I hope she's not like the secretary friend of Carla's. When we were alone in her trailer and she was giving me the tour of her bedroom, I don't know what scared me more – the pink curtains with little kittens or the baby zucchinis on her bedside table." They both laughed at the image.

"I keep telling you, no concepts, my friend. I think that city life and the Maloney baloney is changing you into some anal-retentive Republican or something. Loosen up."

"Then you'll be pleased to hear I'm seriously considering ending my business relationship with Malone, 'cause I suspect he's ripping off the company. I'm not a hundred percent sure but it's only a matter of time before he messes up."

"Finally. Now you're talking, but I wouldn't wait."

"I need to see if I am over-dramatizing the situation because I'm missing out on my writing."

"Stick to getting some good words out to the people, instead of supporting a crook."

"That's the plan, man."

"Just to say, brother, you look like you're starting to turn into some kinda LA cowboy. I can tell you the world ain't all tinsel and bright lights. Don't need to ride off into the sunset to write your story." He was surveying Stephan's outfit like it was a costume: cowboy shirt, large belt buckle and square-toed boots.

"Yes indeed, the maya is thick as a costal fog down there," Stephan answered in acknowledgement of his rock star styling. "Thanks for the reminder, man."

"Can I let you in on a little secret?" Greg asked retrieving a pot from the cupboard. Stephan said 'yeah' and Greg explained how he had hidden some of his money, buying a small property at a remote location about an hour north of San Francisco. He suggested Stephan camp out in the small cabin and make it his writer's retreat for a couple months of distraction-free writing. It was the only way he could see Stephan making any real progress on what Greg saw as his important project and true calling. Stephan was reluctant, as his entanglements wouldn't let him go at the moment so Greg said the offer would always be there. And in another roundabout way to tempt Stephan back north was the promise that the property would become the ultimate yoga center they had talked about so much called Rancho Nirvana. Stephan was touched by his friend's vision and it gave him hope that Greg would eventually find his way back to his true roots as well as let him and Greg recapture the dream that had gotten lost.

Greg was moving from one side of the kitchen to another as he fussed with pots and making room on the stove. "Yes, we're like vampires: getting up when the sun goes down and going to bed when the sun comes up. Ain't much going on anyway until nighttime, so no sense wasting a good night I say. Now that you're here, maybe we should do some asanas."

Greg grabbed a tube of aluminum foil lying nearby and pretending it was flute. He struck a Krishna pose, with one foot tucked into the opposite upper leg, while he trilled some notes, jumping around on one foot, sticking his chin out repeatedly like a chicken on the run and then starting to chant, "Hari Krishna, Hari Krishna, Hari Rama, Rama, Rama," like the cymbal clanging, bald-headed monks on street corners, before stumbling back to two feet, laughing.

Cruising in the Pinto Stephan had borrowed from his dad, Stephan was at the wheel as Greg had seemed less interested in driving these days. Stephan didn't mind being the driver, because on the last visit when they had been going down a backcountry road, Greg's Dodge had suddenly swerved, barely missing the ditch. Greg claimed there had been a squirrel in the road he was trying to avoid, but Stephan knew he had either nodded off or hallucinated.

They had gone to find the girl Greg promised would be Stephan's next soul mate in a run-down neighborhood south of the harbor. Greg had his mile-a-minute rap going about the possibilities of life, a canvas as broad as the known universe, ready to be painted with whatever colors suited one's fancy. He was always bringing the focus back to the endless beauty of creation and the goddess-like creatures populating the planet, clearly intent upon setting up Stephan with a date. Greg wound up his sales pitch with: "And she has one of those high, fine asses like a black chick – megabooty!"

His earlier attempts to fix Stephan up with local girls were well intended but had no results. The prospective ladies had ranged from the hairdresser with Rubenesque endowments who lived in a trailer park and kept vegetable helpers by her bedside to Carla the stripper. Carla had made her offer to sleep with Stephan while the crew (including her boyfriend Jim) were all together in a restaurant loaded on vodka tonics and casually passing around a nasal spray bottle that was filled with water and cocaine.

While buzzed on the coke and a few vodkas, Stephan was so disoriented he didn't know if Carla's offer was a joke or else just one more round of free-living game playing (her boyfriend was also encouraging the act). Stephan declined in a gentlemanly fashion, with a generous 'thanks' and then wondered if he had missed the chance of a lifetime given Carla's dancer body and obvious experience in seduction techniques.

The girl they picked up was blond and pretty, maybe twenty with an outfit from K-mart: tight jeans made out of cheap denim and shoes with thick plastic wedges for heels. As soon as she was in the car and introduced, she asked for a hit. They hadn't moved from the dirt sidewalk, where the car was parked in front of a row of derelict houses with broken porches and weedy yards with dried-up flowerbeds. She was already rolling up her sleeve in the passenger seat.

From the backseat Greasy said, "No worries, baby, we take care of our own." He instructed Stephan to drive to the end of the street where they could park by an empty lot.

Stephan was shocked, but thought it would be hypocritical to tell Greg what to do. Stephan was no paragon of virtue with his welcome embrace of Southern California hedonism, but compared to Greg he was a model of good behavior. Perhaps the role of a straight-ahead existence is what Greg wanted to perpetuate in Stephan because he had never offered Stephan the chance to shoot up, and this was the first time Stephan had seen anyone get a fix.

Greg quickly and expertly prepared a syringe of heroin in a ritual that would have rivaled a Japanese tea ceremony, while Stephan tried chatting with the girl. First the needle was screwed on the syringe and laid out on the top of one leg. A spoon sat on the other and Greg tapped into it a pile of light brown powder out of a small cellophane envelope. He put away the paper and from a small vial of water added a few drops in the spoon. He lit a match under the mix until it slowly bubbled. Greg borrowed a cigarette from the girl and broke off the filter, drawing the mix through it to trap any impurities.

As a substitute for a tourniquet, Greasy instructed Stephan to squeeze the girl's arm above the elbow to get the vein to stand out. Stephan, who anyway hated the sight of needles and was repulsed by the thought of helping someone shoot up, had looked away at the last minute and the spike missed the vein, landing in the muscle when the pressure was inadvertently released by his lack of participation. The girl cursed Greg because she really wanted the rush from mainlining, not the slow buzz of a muscle bang. She was almost in tears, saying it was clear Stephan wasn't into this scene.

They ended up at a run-down bar in the industrial area north of town, where the Coast Highway crawls on its knees out of Santa Cruz and Greg left them discreetly alone with a vodka and tonic each to get acquainted. He borrowed Stephan's car keys to take care of some business in the parking lot, most likely a jab and a nod.

They lost the girl a few hours later in a blur of bar-hopping around town that progressed like sleepwalking through a snowstorm of thick drifts, that made progress heavy and visibility near zero, with faces fading in and out, framed by snatches of glowing conversation that floated by unheard. They found the birthday party, navigating across the city, through the freakish blur of neon signs and winking taillights. Greg's assessment was correct – reality was relative to one's perception. If one were intoxicated enough, then the country singer with the famous boobs like watermelons was really there, because the two brothers had show business connections in Atlantic City and plenty of money. Who was to say if it was the real entertainer or not? The brothers were playing it cool and perhaps bluffing, but the effect was challenging especially after someone handed Stephan a joint of local skunkweed. One puff turned the whole pulsating crowd into an outer space bar scene, like in the movie *Star Wars*, and reality wasn't relevant anymore.

After Greg and Stephan's walk through the doorway between the worlds of perceived and actual reality, the morning arrived too fast. Stephan climbed off the sofa around one, woken by an aching head, hardly remembering how he got there. He knew Greasy was around, because the distinctive wide black leather belt with Spanish buckle lay folded over Stephan's shoes in the hallway, in a gesture of protection.

Jim showed up an hour later for a breakfast of toasted Wonder Bread smeared with margarine and a mug of instant coffee. Jim was stocky and solid, wearing a checked shirt looking every part the roughneck carpenter he worked as from time to time. As soon as Greg and Stephan had revived, Jim, who was having trouble sitting still, said, "Okay, troops, time for a little toot."

"What are you offering?" Greg asked.

"The breakfast of champions, a little China White."

Stephan didn't look too happy, so Jim said, "What's the matter, you never tried this before or what?"

"Can't say that I have," Stephan said with a tone that indicated he also wasn't interested. He was propped on his elbows on the linoleum covered kitchen table and looked into his coffee getting his appetite up with the smell of toasted bread slowly filling the kitchen.

"Look, it ain't no big deal. You won't turn into junkie from just one line," Greg said. "Remember the British fought opium wars with China to make sure they would have a regular supply. Wasn't always illegal, you know. And the original Coca-Cola had cocaine it. Much more enlightened times." Greg was manning the toaster and flipping bread onto plates like a cook in a diner.

"Yeah, and anyone using serious pain relievers has tried synthetic heroin and been grateful for it. Hell, I'm even going to work later this morning," Jim said. "C'mon, just one little line. Make you a mellow fellow." He looked at Stephan with a look of encouragement like it wasn't anything to worry about.

Jim took a plate from the cupboard and laid it on the table. Taking out a tiny plastic bag from his shirt pocket, he tapped a pile of light brown powder onto the plate and started chopping the heroin up with a one-edged razor blade he had in his wallet. Jim scraped together three fat lines out of the pile, about an inch and a half long.

Greg was already hovering around, rolling up a one-dollar bill into a tube. He handed it to Stephan and said, "You'll never know what you're missing, until you try."

Stephan thought he could maintain some credibility with Greg if he knew what Greg's fascination was all about. He had almost lost his street credentials on the last trip, when he was cruising with the two misfits. Greg had put a flake of pure cocaine the size of a pinhead on the back of his hand for Stephan to sniff up. No matter how hard he tried, Stephan couldn't vacuum it up, not being a pro at it, so Jim had quickly maneuvered over, deftly sniffing the alkaloid crumb up his nose.

Sitting in the quiet kitchen, Stephan had a sense of dread. When Jim gave him a hearty slap on the back like they were the best of buddies, Stephan resigned himself to the situation. He bent over the plate with the tubular dollar and sniffed half a line up each nostril to a chorus of "way to go" with the two others quickly following his lead.

There was a brief wave of nausea and then… mellowness. Everything was fine, just fine. The two colleagues were his oldest and dearest comrades and life a wonderful glowing existence. Ahhhh, yes! Or maybe it was only Ohhh, yeah…

row your boat slowly down the stream, life is just a dream. Ummm, a waking softness, as cozy as if you were still under the covers feeling comfortable and safe, while the world appeared vibrant and friendly.

Stephan didn't feel that there was anything special but had he injected it and a wave of instant, intense euphoria permeated his body, the impression would have been different. Maybe he was already too laid back from following a yogic lifestyle, that a dose of mellowness from an opium poppy didn't jolt his awareness. But it was clear why the experience was desirable and eventually addictive.

Now that he was a member of the gang, Greg and Jim drove Stephan over to a garage with some wrecks in the backyard to show off a special car before Jim went off to work. The auto they came to point out was a new model Ford sedan that had the driver's side riddled with bullets like it had been used for target practice. Jim was proud to point out that the car was shot up in front of the owner's house in a nearby quiet suburban street by a semi-automatic rifle one recent evening, but stopping short of naming the shooter.

"Imagine what your neighbors are going to think about you, once you get your car shot to hell. Doesn't say a lot for the type of people you associate with or the line of business you're in," Jim noted. Six months earlier, Stephan had gone with Greg to the same house and had a beer, but now a business associate had become an enemy. Seeing the potential danger, Stephan realized the mysterious wall Greg had mentioned bumping up against in his transactions must have been the local Mafia, which only made him worry more about his friend's long-term survival possibilities.

Stephan had to finally admit there was nothing he could do to positively influence Greg, short of moving to Santa Cruz and that wasn't an option, so a sense of resignation took hold. There was no penetrating Greg's upbeat jive talking long enough to have a serious conversation. Even when they had candidly discussed the situation, Greg admitted he was aware of his drug use, confessing revealingly he had nothing else much going on. He claimed it was only a phase, with something new along the way down the road sure to take its place. Stephan had encouraged him by suggesting he start with a simple step like getting a job again in a garage. Then maybe go to night school and get a degree in counseling, as his people skills and natural supportive style would lend itself to this type work. Greg had listened, finding wisdom in the advice by agreeing to the plan. As he left, Stephan was sure the project would soon be forgotten without anyone to walk Greg through the necessary steps and keep him focused. He remembered what James had said to him a few months earlier that junkies are programmed to tell you want you want to hear.

Greg's parting words were like a benediction, reminding Stephan that life could offer sweet seductions but the universe rewarded those who remembered the true nature of things. He finished with, "Write that book, boy!"

On the return trip over the hill, Stephan reflected on his latest adventure. The heroin he tried was only a token amount and he certainly wasn't feeling like he needed or wanted another dose, in the short or long term. He felt he had betrayed Greg, by endorsing the one thing that was slowly killing his friend. Condoning its use by accepting a hit and helping a young girl to shoot up, he had lost the aura of saintliness (if ever he really had one) that Greg associated with him. Any leverage that was empowered by representing the counter-point was lost.

Why make any more trips north to help with a detox when at the end you join the cured individual by indulging in the source of the pain? Was Stephan an enemy or a friend? What had become of the brotherhood of seekers of truth? Stephan kicked himself for again acting unconsciously. The path was straight and narrow, but now Stephan was sure he had lost his way and didn't know where to turn anymore. If he could accept supporting people to get lost in the illusions of this world and ultimately be a partner to their self-destruction, his inspired living was as superficial as the shabby facades he had dragged around sound stages. And now returning to LA he was afraid where his compromised moral nature would lead him. And to add to his wall of writer's block was ten tons of stone in the form of self-doubt for his writing to be able to have the authenticity of a person with idealistic values. He wondered how and if he could recover his sense of pride and purpose or even if he had it left in him to find a way to try and reach out again, offering a hand to a fallen friend.

17

SHIFTING SANDS

With his fear of snakes that originated in India when he had to dodge stray cobras in the wild, Stephan was watching for any coiled-up reptiles in the shady areas of the arroyo where he and Roscoe were jogging. Stephan was getting an extra adrenaline rush every time he saw the wispy 'S' shaped trails from a sidewinder where it had crawled over a sand bank forming the side of the dry streambed. That particular venomous snake's sneaky sideways movement earned it the name that described how you never knew which way it was going to strike.

They were having an early morning jog through the desert before the heat got too oppressive, planning their week's game. It was more like a fast walk as Roscoe was already puffing from the exertion of tying his running shoes.

"You know, Stephan, this operation is going to be big. I'm already going to expand the imitation leather shoe line to include distributing Earth Shoes."

Stephan didn't look convinced; he had been an early adopter, owning a pair of the clunky looking shoes from Sweden. They had a wide front end to give space to the toes and a lower heel area, so the overall effect was like walking in sand to appeal to those seeking a natural posture with better alignment of the spine. They were sold as 'walking yoga'.

"I don't know. The ones I owned gave me blisters. Besides that, they're ugly."

"Well, now they've improved the design. It's all about synergy, my friend. I'm even talking with a guy south of the border about making quality huaraches. No retreads, only original tires with good profile for the sole. I tell you, the natural shoe market is going to be huge."

"I've got some new cover ideas from the designer for the tantra and the betting books. She even came up with a concept for your wealth creation project."

"It's crap, all crap. A seven-year-old child could do better than that," Malone snapped.

"I thought the tantra design had a good balance between the Indian flavor and hint of sensuality, without being vulgar," Stephan said as he methodically plodded through the loose sand grinding underfoot.

"I was thinking we should put together a line of flavored massage oils to go with the book. Create a brand around it. Lady Bluffington is such a character we can market everything from bedroom play toys to trashy lingerie. I want you to see who makes the oils and if we can lock up the rights. Has to be edible, with natural colors." Malone was slowing down and wiped his sweaty forehead on a sleeve of his shirt.

"Maybe we should get the book published first," Stephan said.

"Why don't you get the designer started on the gambling

book? You're creative – give her a brief. That's the one which will make us some fast bucks."

"Why don't we get one design completed first and then go on to the next? With all this back and forth on projects, she's talking about heading back to LA. She doesn't think we're focused or have enough work for her beyond next month." Stephan was staring ahead partly looking for snake trails but more to contain his anger. He was sure if he looked at Malone he would start an argument he couldn't win.

"Screw her, there's always another one."

They had slowed to a walk as the conversation had winded Malone. Stephan was getting frustrated trying to defend his ideas for the publishing business, knowing he would always be outranked because Malone was the CEO of the holding company. The warm wind smelling of sage and creosote was blowing towards Las Vegas and momentarily kicked up swirls of dust, getting grit in their eyes.

"Roscoe, there's something else. The two accounts in LA at the TV station and non-profit outfit aren't going to renew their newsletter contracts with us. They say we're not responsive enough because we're too far away now."

"I'll go have a word with those sons-of-bitches next time I'm in town."

"Last time you were meant to see them you spaced it out. And the time before that, you severely pissed them off. I've been getting these calls complaining about our charges. And when I looked at the bills you sent them, there were some materials listed I didn't know we had." They were marching in step now like two disciplined soldiers each intent on their goal of finishing the drill.

"What's the problem? They can afford it."

"Maybe I should go have a talk with them to keep the peace. Is everything okay with you? Something up between you and Hart?"

"No problemo, amigo. You think you can handle them better, then do it." Malone sounded both hurt and scornful. "Hart and I are as happy as can be, don't worry. And if those outfits don't renew, you can use the extra time to help out with the arcade. I just bought a couple more of those Space Invaders machines to put in that old gas station on Main Street."

"Those games are really a blast but I need time to get on with my book."

"Don't sweat it. These video arcades are money machines, I tell you. Big stuff, huge. Going to call this business Electrotainment Studios. With this company in our corporate family we will have the diversity to make us a juicy takeover candidate. Hang onto your shares, boy; we're all going to be rich. Know what I'm going to do with my money?"

"No idea."

"Start the whole story over again and find me some distressed companies or underdeveloped niche markets to make another monster corporation out of."

Unknown to anyone, Malone's fragmented approach was now being enhanced by little lines of white powder that were secretly finding their way up his nose. Roscoe hid his use because he knew that if Hart found out she would make a scene. There had been too many war stories from the rock world about damaged lives from the cocaine epidemic that was spreading far and wide.

What started as a flurry had developed into a blizzard and hit the town of glamour and glitter with conspicuous consumption rampant. The signs were starting to pop up everywhere – long lines at parties to get in the bathroom, pictures off the walls lying around on tables, small vanity mirrors scattered about even in men's apartments, cut-down McDonald's plastic soda straws from handfuls grabbed while getting a burger.

Then there was the chopping sound of razors on glass, the scratching rasp of lines being drawn out of the freshly fluffed-up mound of powder, red sniffling noses with sores on the inside edge from where the straw had rubbed too much, rapping of small brown bottles to empty their contents onto hard surfaces followed by the repetitive, patient clacking as the rocks and chunks got broken down with the delicate whine of the blade against glass as the powder feathered into a long line with a long exaggerated sniff while one nostril is pinched closed (a Western style of yoga breathing) and the line is vacuumed up; or the quick, deep sharp sniff from a miniature spoon, ladies with little fingernails narrowed for perfect dipping and scooping, keys getting jabbed into bottles or folded-up small squares of white pharmaceutical paper or glossy magazine covers as well as Bic pen tops with their narrow pocket clip extending from the cap, perfectly shaped to dip and 'flick my Bic'.

The sight of greasy mirrors where the tooters had

wiped their fingers over the dust left by the line hoping for a few crumbs more to rub on their gums for a Novocain effect was a common scene. The clean chemical smell and antiseptic semi-bitter taste dripping down the back of the throat accompanied bags of mannite and baby laxative to dilute the mix. People talking a mile a minute in the most meaningful conversations they had ever known. There were dancing fools, friends being ripped off by friends and frantic midnight calls looking for one more toot. Instant lifelong friends who suddenly appear out of nowhere when a little white powder is produced, itchy noses and rolled up dollar bills at the ready.

The joke around town was that people were so desperate for the drug they were sniffing the white lines off the freeway.

The deceptive nature of Malone's drug use also created an invisible barrier between him and Stephan that wasn't noticeable at first, but whose presence became slowly felt. Maybe it was something to do with all the 'private phone calls' that had to be made from behind closed doors and frequent trips to the bathroom in the middle of meetings.

Malone tried to keep his secret use of coke hidden from Stephan in case he was seen to be appropriating company money and being generally irresponsible. It was the perfect drug for a high-powered executive to reinforce the image in his own mind of his greatness and the incredible genius of the ideas that popped up after a quick snort. Negotiations would be easier when the mind was primed with a sniff of powder that led to quick thinking and witty repartee.

But an already exaggerated ego enhanced with the powder of dreams meant that Malone felt he didn't need anyone's help because he was all-powerful, keen of insight and true in action, so one by one partnerships started to unravel.

The first one to go was with the New York publisher Stephan had lined up to license the *Star Sign Calendar* under their own imprint, retaining Malone and him as the author and editor. The deal was close to completion but Malone laughed at the contract and berated the larger company's junior executive so much the deal got pulled, frustrating Stephan who had spent many months building the relationship and shaping the contract. If they had pulled it off there were even talks of being a boutique imprint of the larger parent, creating original titles and having a huge organization to back them up. Stephan had also been hoping that with an eventual connection with a publisher it would allow him to get his Rama story into print.

The next contract to fall by the wayside was with their distributor who had taken the *Star Sign Calendar* into most bookshops in California. In an effort to save from the bottom line, the percentage the distributor took from the sales, Malone wanted Stephan to load up the trunk and backseat of his car with calendars and become a traveling salesman, directly supplying the bookstores that carried last year's calendar.

Stephan tried to explain that with the loan money it was better to build up the catalog of Great Impressions and leave the drudgework like schlepping calendars to the distributor who did it anyway. The plea fell on deaf ears so the calendar looked like it was going to be a one-season wonder after last year's phenomenal growth, as Stephan didn't see himself going door-to-door up and down the state.

Frustrated and angry, Stephan was leaving the desert office one day when an older man in an expensive double-breasted grey suit with an open shirt and greased-back hair, who looked like he shaved with a broken bottle, stopped him in the doorway and asked him curtly, "Is this dump Malone's office?"

"That's right. His desk is through that door, in the back," Stephan said pointing across the room.

Malone heard the conversation and came to his office door. "Mr. Gotti, welcome to my empire."

"Empire, shit! Where's my goddamn money from the oil wells, you fucking shyster."

"I was just cutting you the next dividend check. Come on in." Stephan watched them disappear into Malone's office, guessing that the loan money wasn't all going to the business. Outside, a dust-covered Cadillac with Nevada license plates took up two parking spaces next to their building and a squat man in a cheap black nylon windbreaker and wraparound shades leaned against the front fender having a cigarette, giving Stephan a stare that was chilly even in the desert heat.

On his visits to LA Stephan would stay on Mac's sofa, acting as script editor and sympathetic set of ears, discussing plot revisions on the screenplay project and the modest, infrequent progress on his own novel. Each time he returned he was increasingly torn between his desert identity and giving it all up to move back to LA. Even though he had sublet his Blem cabana he could have it back on short notice as the tenant, a friend of the band, was mostly at his girlfriend's place anyway.

"Sounds to me like a case of the Emperor's new clothes, where only the Emperor believes he is the best-dressed man in the kingdom," Mac said. He and Stephan were sitting on the front porch of Mac's place, having a coffee in the morning sun.

Stephan went on to explain that after Malone screwed up the publishing deals and the graphics crew drifted off, he had tried to assure Stephan that what was good for the parent corporation was good for the publishing business. Unfortunately, the circumstances were getting suspicious. And without the extra income from working on film productions, Stephan was entirely dependent on the company's fortunes to pay his living expenses.

"What about the loan money, I thought you had a big pile for the publishing biz?" Mac enquired.

Stephan told about how the loans that were being pooled into a common pot to support all the businesses and as a result the publishing business was getting cash-starved, including the paltry salary he was being paid. Also, large amounts of money seemed to be disappearing without any bills or receipts to explain it. The small amount of money that found its way to the calendar resulted in a better cover but the other aspects of the project were hanging. Stephan felt very vulnerable because he was dependent on Malone. At the same time, he was increasingly nervous about his association with Malone because as a business partner he could be held accountable for the loan money. More frightening were the clients of the oil futures business who looked at him as an accomplice in the shady scheme.

"One step forward, ten steps back."

Reedo came out of his bungalow bleary-eyed and ragged, looking for the paper. He called out: "Hey, guys, what's up?" He wearily scooped up the *LA Times*, freeing it from the rubber band that held it in a roll and wandered over in his pajama bottoms and famous hair looking like a scarecrow that had been attacked by a flock of birds. He still smelled like the Hai Karate he bathed in before a night out.

"We're just getting ready for the next round of bashing the script together. Is my song number one yet?" Stephan said as Reedo leaned on the railing alongside the steps for support.

"I wish it were so," he said in a tired voice, trying to surface to the reality of a new morning. "Right now we have to fight for every dime we can to get any promotion. Jack calls the label almost every day. At least it looks like we have another tour coming up. Until then, I'm the Mac's drum roadie."

"Cool. Get ready for them groupies," Stephan said.

"I made a scoring system for chicks. Maximum is one hundred points. Each girl can get a possible twenty-five points for each section from top to bottom: face, tits, ass and legs," Reedo said switching to his favorite topic.

"What about brains?" Maceo asked as he stretched his legs out down the porch stairs.

"If the visuals don't work it doesn't matter if she's a

rocket scientist. Know what I mean?" Reedo let go of the railing and glanced at the headlines in the paper he was holding.

"I would have thought having a conversation with more than mono-syllable words would be important," Stephan said.

"Sure, my last lady was like that but she went and broke my heart by going her own way. We were perfect." Reedo looked at Stephan with a hangdog look of lost love.

"You mean the designer girl with the boutique?" Stephan asked.

"Yeah. She's Stevie Nicks's best friend. When I do gigs with the band we see each other, but it's real painful."

"Don't give up, love will find a way," Stephan said.

"I had a date last night. This bird I know from the Valley. You should have seen her. We were in this restaurant and I made sure she was under the air-con. Her nipples stuck out like nose cones on a rocket." Everyone laughed and Reedo smiled at the memory as he wandered off to his bungalow.

Malone's drug use finally came to light when Stephan bumped into The Count later that afternoon. Maceo had just left for a late shift of filling planes for the airlines when Harry showed up, and while the two of them shared a beer getting mellow behind some Steely Dan jazzy rock tunes, Harry asked Stephan about life in the desert.

"How's my favorite desert doll Sid doing?" Harry asked from where he sat at Maceo's desk looking down on Stephan lying back on the futon sofa.

"I think she misses you. Every time I see her she asks

where you are," Stephan said with a grin, leading Harry on.

"Get out of here. She really said that? I need to visit her soon, I guess." Harry wasn't too sure if Stephan was joking or not and had hopes he was serious.

"She said she named her vibrator Harry."

"Fuck you." They both laughed and Harry reached over and they clinked beers.

"You're missing some great parties, that's for sure," Stephan said.

"When you heading back out there?" Harry asked as he looked around at the books scattered on the worktable.

"Tomorrow afternoon."

"Want to take along an eighth for your partner?"

"For Roscoe?!"

"Oops, maybe I wasn't supposed to let you know."

Stephan masked his surprise to not offend Harry and also so he could get a little more information. "No, it's cool. He shares everything. I'm just surprised because he always says someone at the studio gave him the coke he uses."

"Yeah, well you know it's not all for him."

"Do tell." Stephan asked, curious.

"Seems he has a thing going on with a lady we all know." Harry looked at Stephan with a sly smile.

"Let me guess. Zoomer – as in our former secretary?"

"Nope. Getting warm. Keep guessing," The Count said taking a swallow from his beer.

"Lady Bluffington, the tantra queen?" Stephan guessed.

"Warmer…"

"Holy Shit, you mean Sinful Cindee?" Stephan sat up

and looked at The Count with disbelief.

"Burning hot! You got it, brother. Seen them heading into the Les Hot Tub Club one night after I sold him a gram. Sporting around in one of the Malibu rock star's wheels that got saved and stored in a garage – the little Benz."

Stephan suddenly realized where all the loan money was going which didn't bode well for the longevity of the publishing company. "I guess I shouldn't ask too many questions."

"Look, I don't want to get mixed up in the middle of your business arrangements."

"Don't worry, this doesn't involve you. We never had this conversation," Stephan said casually to wind down the discussion.

"Cool, I appreciate that."

Stephan masked his shock with his dispassionate yogi attitude while inside he was fuming. Cindee was one of a series of temporary secretaries that helped out on the Globall Corporations various activities, replacing an earlier one called Zoomer (the ultimate Zuma Beach babe) who had moved along to a PR outfit. Lady Bluffington had introduced Cindee to the company when she brought her along to an editorial meeting. They had both been on Bob Dylan's Rolling Thunder tour more or less in the capacity of groupies and extras in the psuedo-documentary that was getting filmed en route. Cindee had that slinky style of low-slung jeans and loose T-shirt that seemed ready to fall off in the slightest breeze. Combined with deep green sleepy eyes and long, thick hair, she had an allure that men found irresistible.

Being out of touch with Cindee after the move to the desert when her help was no longer required, Stephan had thought she had left LA and gone back to the east coast but apparently, he was wrong. Stephan wasn't sure how to use Harry's information, and even with his intent to make things work, his will was being challenged as he felt increasingly like a fool and at the same time feeling sorry for Hart.

That evening before heading back to Desert Hot Springs, Stephan had organized a rare rendezvous with Lila at yoga class and afterward they went to their usual hangout for a meal. Bilkem knew of Stephan's desert expeditions and would always try and set him up with a companion for the weekend by announcing loudly at the end of the class that Stephan was driving out to the desert and had room in his car.

"Did the great yogi find you a desert date?" Lila said. She was sitting opposite Stephan at a two-person table but had her eyes on the door when she spoke.

"I think it's just another one of his jokes. You know, a little taste of a sexual innuendo. Maybe he's being real and wants me to find a nice lady. So why not someone with a similar interest in yoga?" He looked at Lila meaningfully but she ignored his plain stare. Even though she was continuously chasing power people who might get her into a film, Stephan still felt there was a special quality to their relationship, as yet unfulfilled. He knew from their soulful conversations that behind her career girl exterior there was someone more sensitive and able to rise above the crazy world in which she moved.

"Do you know who that was you were talking to after class?" Lila asked.

"No, should I? You mean the lady I was chatting with about the weather."

"Yeah, that was Raquel Welch." Lila took a congratulatory sip of her carrot juice for having known who the person was.

"Really? When she was lying there next to me I was thinking how good it was that these middle-aged housewives get out and take care of themselves."

"You didn't know who it was, really?" Lila blotted her lips with a napkin to make sure she wasn't wearing any orange color from the juice.

"Now that you mention it there was a special something about her when she came out in makeup and a tight dress. Or maybe it was the new Jag she drove off in. I think if she wore her fur bikini from the *One Million Years B.C.* film I would have got it sooner. Maya, maya, my – nothing is as it seems…" Stephan said as he shook his head wistfully.

"Speaking of maya, how's your epic tale coming along?"

"To be honest, I haven't been such a good scribe lately. I'm afraid I'm letting down the silent baba by slacking off on my story." Stephan was picking at his salad trying to separate the ever-present alfalfa sprouts from the rest of the greenery.

"Living a life of truth is never easy… here in the West especially. Don't be so hard on yourself."

"Thanks. That reminds me – there was one thing I came across in my research that reminded me of you." He looked at Lila with a knowing smile.

"Oh, really?" Lila smiled back with a mixture of pride and shyness.

"When Rama finds out where his wife is being held captive, he secretly sends a message to assure her that they will soon be together again and not to worry. It's not only a really beautiful acknowledgement of his love for her, it's also representing the words of a teacher to his student, to express his care and to say keep the faith. Very special."

"And that made you think of me?"

"A lot of things make me think of you. And when I see you in yoga I'm reminded you're not just a pretty face but someone with deeper aspirations in life." There was a short pause as Lila quickly digested the words that had remained unspoken until now.

"Thanks, Mister Spiritually Correct, you're always trying to remind everyone what's really important in life." To deflect that she had been touched by Stephan's words she was playfully sarcastic but the bland tone of her delivery made it less offensive. She smiled shyly and then took a moment to scan the room for A-listers before turning back and avoiding the subject. "Hey, did I tell you I heard about these things called samadhi tanks."

"Like in a holy war?"

"No silly, like a giant bathtub you immerse yourself in that has a cover on it. You're floating in this salty liquid so you're weightless and all your senses become inactive because it's quiet and dark and the liquid is body temperature."

"Like when I meditate."

"It is so cool. I had like an out-of-body experience. And every sensation is magnified. It's like being on mushrooms."

"So every time I want my awareness heightened I have to pay twenty bucks and hope the last person who got in didn't piss in it?"

"Come on, don't be so negative." They both laughed at Stephan's joke.

"I'm just teasing you. I already saw one of those things at Esalen when I was there for a weekend workshop." Lila was scanning the room again casually so Stephan took a chance to further express his feelings towards her. "You should come visit me sometime. The water's amazing, as you know. And if we both looked together for the door to another reality, maybe our combined energies could open it."

"Thanks, you're a sweetheart. I think that would be nice. I'll get back to you on that," Lila said, smiling and leaning over to peck him on the cheek. It temporarily placated Stephan but he was as unsure as ever if there would be a chance for them to get together.

A few days after he returned to the desert Stephan was invited for dinner at the Malones and a surprise guest was waiting. Tania was a friend of the band and a casual acquaintance from the parties in the Silver Lake house a year earlier. She was an attractive blond in her mid-twenties from Arizona who had drifted into LA to handle some business dealings and ended up hanging out with the band after a concert and got to know the boys.

Tania had recently returned from the Philippines where

she had sought psychic treatment for cancer of the liver. The psychic healers were a last resort, but it was unclear if the treatments had been a success. She had been visiting the famous doctors shown in documentaries performing miracle cures, where they could insert their hands into the patient's body without incisions and wrestle the disease away. She had remained hopeful and was planning of visiting some doctors in LA. Her positive spirit gave her an extra measure of energy that kept her going.

Hart was a perfect and gracious hostess and had made an elegant table setting in the dining room with a floral centerpiece surrounded by good china and designer serving dishes. After the main course of vegetarian lasagna had been served Malone thought he would lighten up the semi-formal setting by scratching his belly and stifling belches in an attempt to put the guests at ease as if he were an eccentric host unaware of his bad behavior. Finally, Hart had to say something, effectively ending the show of intentional bad manners because while Tania and Stephan had been ignoring the antics it was visibly getting on Hart's nerves. It slowly became obvious that there was a deeper antagonism behind the scene and it would be better to leave the couple alone to work it out. After dessert Stephan offered to show Tania the famous oasis pool at Two Bunch Palms. Hart and Malone gave their enthusiastic approval as a must-see attraction because the resort was the most exclusive in the area, having hosted the Rolling Stones and most of the big names in Hollywood at one time or another.

Originally the spa was Al Capone's hideaway when he fled Chicago to escape the law. He had sent two of his lieutenants to explore the area around Palm Springs and they had located a small oasis with two large bunches of palms in the middle of nowhere which in their regional dialect got shortened to Two Bunch. The old stone house of Al's was still on the property, lost amongst the bungalows, tennis courts and mud treatment areas. The pool at Two Bunch was surrounded by ancient palm trees and had a rocky landscaping with a small waterfall to make it seem like a native locale rather than the centerpiece of the most expensive spa in town. The edges of the pool had a four-foot-wide shelf about ten inches deep, so guests could lay back with only their head above water, soaking in the healing mineral water and admiring the desert sky through the palm fronds. Stephan knew the back road into the spa the staff used, so they could avoid the security guard at the front gate. This allowed them to slip in without being challenged, as only paying guests were permitted on the property.

The romantic setting and friendly chatter, helped by a mild intoxication from some Zinfandel and mutual needs, slowly worked to bring Stephan and Tania into a passionate coupling. They were lying side-by-side gently talking about their lives, forming a momentary closeness on the shallow shelf in the warm water of the oasis. Tania had an athletic body, nicely accented by a French bikini and in the moonlight her blond hair shimmered like hammered gold. Soon they were embracing and their wet bodies slid together kissing hungrily in a tight embrace. They found a quiet place behind some rocks in a dark, shadowy corner of the pool. Tania eased onto Stephan's lap with her legs wrapped around him to form one pulsating being in a short passionate session of lovemaking.

Neither was sure of the other's ultimate intentions, and being unable or afraid to articulate their feelings, it made for a subdued ride back to the Malone's where Stephan dropped Tania off rather than invite her over to his place for the night.

Stephan sat out in the backyard when he got home downing beers, wondering about what had happened. Stephan knew that Tania was in a fragile state due to her cancer and wanted to be respectful of her needs but wasn't sure how to proceed. He was unable to take it for what it was, a one-night stand and a roundabout act of caring, and started feeling guilty. Too many conflicting emotions and impressions collided in the front of his brain in a swirl of thoughts including images of Lila. Stephan had always liked to believe that he needed a deep heartfelt love to have an intimate encounter with real meaning. Using someone just to satisfy basic lusts didn't sit comfortably with him and cheapened the encounter according to his overly intellectual understanding of love and passion. Stephan had intended for his life to reflect correct actions but he seemed to be going backwards lately in his personal evolution. Then he remembered Greg's counsel, when he said Stephan thought about things too much, acting like a priest (which in part echoed some of Lila's comments). Maybe Greg was right, life was for living and was flying by too fast not to enjoy.

In the cool of the morning Stephan sat outside his trailer absorbing the tranquil desert landscape as the early morning sun painted rose highlights on the foothills, contemplating his situation while a cup of Morning Thunder tea eased his hangover. The sun was still too low on the horizon to make it hot and high overhead a convoy of helicopters flew over towards the Marine Corps base in Twentynine Palms behind the foothills of the western boundary of Joshua Tree, a mile from his trailer. He closed his eyes attempting to sit quietly and remember a few breaths going in and out to try and focus his conflicting emotions to get at the heart of the matter.

Finally, he drove over to the local bank located in a humble brick building along a stretch of the main road leading out of town. He parked in a sand-covered parking lot next to a pile of tumbleweeds quivering in the morning breeze. The wind in this end of the Coachella Valley never stopped reshaping nature, which is why it was less developed than Palm Springs. He needed to pick up some cash for gas and expenses but had a rude awakening when the teller told him the balance in the Great Impressions account was only twelve dollars and eighty-five cents. He headed straight over to the Globall offices on the main street and found Malone in his office bashing out some correspondence on the typewriter.

"Roscoe, can we talk?" Stephan asked coolly, without any greeting, standing in the doorway.

"Sure. What's up?" Roscoe answered without looking up from his hunt and peck attempt at writing a letter, as the round silver ball on the IBM Selectric rotated and smacked on his paper hesitantly.

"I just went by the bank and they said the publishing

account is empty. How is that possible? There was at least ten grand in there a week ago."

Roscoe stopped his writing and turned to Stephan. "I had to transfer some of the money to the other company accounts to keep them going. What's good for one company is good for them all."

"I don't get it."

"As you know, the plan is to build up the corporation's assets so that it can be sold off. And you as president of Great Impressions will be rewarded handsomely. The sum is equal to the parts, so all the units need to be operating at a profit. The publishing business is doing well but I needed a little help for the mail order business to cover some inventory bills."

"We were supposed to get another check for five thou last week," Stephan said with his words taking on a confronting tone.

"We did. You weren't around so I transferred the money," Malone casually replied as he pulled the paper out of the typewriter.

"What are you talking about? You forged my name and took the money?" Stephan was starting to get angry as he saw he was being played for a fool.

"Hey, slow down. Remember we're partners. All the money we receive goes into one pot and we manage the expenses from there." Malone was ignoring him as he studied the letter he had just typed.

"What am I supposed to live off of – my bills were paid out of that account. And I'm going to LA in a couple of hours."

"Look, I'll give you some cash from the video game business to hold you over." Malone looked at him trying to sound friendly and businesslike.

"I'm not sure I like this arrangement of robbing Peter to pay Paul. And as far as any potential rewards, I'd feel a lot more comfortable if I had that in writing."

"Come on, we're like brothers. If you can't trust me who can you trust?" The phrase echoed in a distant corner of Stephan's brain, reminding him briefly of the hustlers in India trying to make their deals saying they wouldn't even give their brother such a good price. Roscoe pulled open the bottom desk drawer beside his chair and took out a small, green metal cash box. He counted out two hundred in twenties and made a notation in a receipt book.

Stephan took the money, mumbled thanks and stormed out. He was trembling with anger but his self-imposed ideal of calm and detachment held him back from exploding in front of Malone like a part of him wanted to. Instead he crunched his gearshift into reverse without much thought to working the clutch and sped over to the trailer to pick up his gear.

Adding to Stephan's sense of frustration was his knowledge of what Malone was doing on the sly in LA and he was unable to confront him on this issue, as it would compromise his promise to Harry. Also, out of respect to Hart who had been kind to him, he didn't want to be the one to bring the bad news of Roscoe's philandering. He decided it would be better for them to sort it out between themselves, even though it was probably wrong to stay quiet.

Stephan sat at the counter in his modular Formica-covered kitchen and had a cup of coffee thinking about his situation. He knew what Malone was doing with the money was incorrect, but he had no other option than to stick it out and trust that Malone would see the rickety ship to the promised golden shore. His doubts were growing, and by being tied up with Malone and a named owner of the publishing business he had to salvage what he could. He promised himself that he would use the trip to drum up some more business and push the people producing the betting and massage books to finish their endless works in progress to add to the income prospects. His rationalization calmed him down enough to start his trek. He didn't get to the question of acceptance – being able to admit he had made a mistake in this partnership and it was better to leave and cut his losses.

Stephan's next challenge was how to avoid Tania, because she was going to LA that morning and would stay overnight at Jack and Reedo's. He decided to delay his return trip until she had left rather than make a caravan with their two cars. And yet while Stephan felt momentarily relieved to be rid of any attachment and resulting support for Tania, a sense of guilt dogged him for the next few weeks. This was accentuated because he genuinely liked Tania, the easy laugh, the friendly smile and simple conversation. Besides that, she also looked amazing in her pink bikini. And yet, knowing she was terminally ill confused him because he had never been in this situation before and didn't know how to find the balance of friendship and caring while not wanting her becoming dependent on him. Unsure of how to further deal with the situation, he avoided Tania at the couple of parties that followed the band's local club appearances and inconspicuously slipped in and out of Maceo's bungalow.

After brooding at Maceo's for many evenings, Stephan stopped his self-indulgent beer consumption and started spending afternoons at the Lake Retreat, the park built by the famous yogi named Yogananda back in the 1920s at the end of Sunset Boulevard, where it ended at the ocean. The tranquil setting of a small lake, surrounded by exotic trees reinforced his higher aspirations. He was also working his way with renewed vigor through the Ramayana, as he dug back into his writing inspired by being around Mac. He was trying to work through his frustrations by focusing on ultimately what he saw as his higher purpose.

One afternoon Stephan was sitting at a café by the beach in Venice having a beer with Maceo while watching the skaters and freaks parade by.

"With this kind of a circus how can anyone like us expect to come up with a more colorful story," Stephan said.

"Maybe it's safer living in our imagination. I don't want to think what would happen if we took a couple of those skater girls home with us." They both laughed as another long-legged blond in cut-off jeans and a bikini top sailed by doing some ballerina moves.

"Sitting here is like getting the inspiration from a hundred muses for the price of a brew," Stephan said taking a sip from his beer.

"Maybe it helps your story but I don't see how those

babes relate to an astronaut."

"Sure they do – they're from another planet where an alternative reality exists. Just like with Malone, the normal rules don't apply."

"From what you told me about that guy you're better off cutting your losses and moving on. Seriously."

"I'm guessing it's my pacifist side holding me back when what I really need to do is get righteously pissed off."

"That's what I'm telling you." Mac took a swig of beer and put the bottle down hard on the table to emphasize his point.

"The whole scene with Tania threw me off balance. Made me realize I should be more caring and respectful."

"So show her some love and give Malone the finger. It's clearly an issue for you. There's the balance you're looking for. Just go find the girl and be her friend. The Malone bullshit you can deal with later."

"Thanks, buddy; I'll do that." Stephan smiled in acknowledgement and they clinked beer bottles, took a last swig and moved along. An ever-present local denizen, a black guy with an electric guitar dressed in something between yoga whites and an Arabic costume complete with turban and over-sized sunglasses, swung in a circle on his skates and parked nearby to play for change.

With his feelings clarified and made strong, Stephan went looking for Tania to be honest with her and offer his friendship, while apologizing for his selfish mistreatment. Stephan caught Jack at home that evening after he and the band had returned from a small concert tour to San Diego and asked where Tania was staying. Jack was somber for a minute and told him he was too late – she had passed away five days earlier.

Stephan was stunned by the news and didn't know what to say. In a state of shock, he went back to his bungalow that he had reclaimed the day before and sat quietly reflecting on the situation, trying to learn what lessons he could. Somewhere in his core he had been touched. This wasn't a scripture or holy book with wise words; this was his life's lesson, a personal instruction just for him, right here, right now.

Nothing had shaken him to his core like the passing of Tania except for the girl being ritually burned in India. Once again he felt like he was standing on the edge of a dark, bottomless abyss with the constricting sense of his finiteness staring him eye to eye, challenging him to take a step. The feelings of despair and helplessness at the inability to change something came back from the scene in India and he felt the same sorrow for the death of another innocent soul that made his eyes hot with tears.

He swore to himself that the Ramayana story would now be a truer expression of his heart, the way he originally envisioned it to be. He also wanted to share this important lesson with his friends up north and perhaps he could reignite that fire they had all felt not so long ago. He also wanted to talk to Greg about his guilt from suggesting a race and work through their mutual issues associated with the cousin's death. Checking in on Greg who was an increasingly lost soul and reminding him of their spiritual roots could help steer him away from disaster and provide a bit more impetus for Stephan as he sought to refocus.

Somehow it was a new stage of awareness, that even though it wasn't the total experience he had sought, it was an important milestone along the way.

Stephan affirmed his resolution to address other issues that he had been handling with similar blindness. The first was his business arrangement with Malone. Now the bridges needed burning and the dream of a desert empire would soon be buried beneath the shifting sands like so many other lost civilizations under the Sahara. It was a dangerous dance, because even if Stephan could break his obligation to continue the business arrangement with Malone, the complicity in using money from the false loan applications meant he shared a criminal act that his partner would not soon let him forget.

18

EVERY CLOUD HAS A GOLDEN LINING

Stephan didn't need a soothsayer translating star signs to know that it was a fortuitous time to think about a career change. The most auspicious pointers were a struggling business that had been built on hype and shifty finances, a tin box trailer in the middle of the desert to call home and a self-centered partner who put federal government loans up his nose. He knew he had to get closure somehow on his relationship with Malone. He recognized it would take courage to leave one dream behind by breaking off their relationship but he also knew that dealing with addicts (Greg included) was a no-win situation. In Greg's case he felt he had a personal stake to help him as a brother but with Malone it was different. He knew he was being used and only more trouble would come of working together. Stephan set up a meeting with Malone at the desert offices on a Friday afternoon and practiced his speech on the two-hour drive down Interstate 10.

The large main room on the first floor of the forgotten looking office building was like one of the abandoned offices at Producers Studio. It had the same dust-covered desks and scattered books and documents that were too useless to waste the energy on of throwing them away. Stale, recycled fumes from an ancient air-conditioner that were meant to cool the room made it smell like a stagnant pond. Malone as usual was on the phone and as Stephan walked back towards Malone's private area the call ended.

"Hi, Roscoe." Stephan greeted Malone but didn't bother to sit down in one of the guest chairs, standing with his arms crossed.

"Stephan, welcome. It's been awhile. What's with the defensive posture – you look like you're protecting yourself with those crossed arms." Malone spoke with an air of superiority, wearing an open neck shirt and suit jacket with a blinding plaid pattern, planting his hands on the edge of his desk in a receptive gesture.

Stephan ignored the comment. "I'll make it very simple 'cause I know you're a busy guy." Malone leaned back in his chair smiling and put his hands behind his head. "I want out. I want my name removed from any and every legal document attaching me to your business."

"Now why would you want to do a thing like that for," Malone drawled. "Great Impressions is more your baby than anyone else's. You will never get another chance like this again. Ever."

"It's not about my dream to make an honorable profession. I've had it with your two-faced behavior and screwy business deals. If you want some fall guy to take a dive for you when everything goes south, you'll have to advertise because I'm out." Stephan stood behind a guest chair and put his hands on the top of the backrest.

"You're accusing me of illegal activities? You better be careful that might be construed as slander." Malone's eyes narrowed like he was preparing to fight.

"Then you can explain it to the same judge you are in front of for all the fake loans you put together."

Malone sat up straight behind the desk. "I'd be careful what you say. You're as much complicit in any loan manipulation as I am by virtue of the fact that you took the money as salary."

"You'll have to prove that but the fact of the matter is that I didn't sign any of your stinking loans. I'm not asking for anything – no materials, no documents, no draft texts. It's over between us."

"You sound serious."

"Look, I don't want to drag this out but if you give me any grief then I will report you to the government for faking the loans. Probably they can't prove anything one way or the other but you'll be on their watch list and a lot more accountable for how you spend the money. If that's what you want, I won't hesitate a second to drop the dime." Stephan squared his shoulders and thrust his hands in his jeans pockets. He was sweating even though the air-conditioner was blowing arctic cold swamp air into the room.

"Okay, calm down. You really want out? No more chance to make your own life? Fine, go back to your manual labor. I don't care. But this isn't about the money, is it?" Malone leaned on his desk and looked at Stephan with a sly smile.

"You're right. It's more about trust and honesty. I don't

think you've been straight with me. And now that we finally have a shot at success, you're screwing things up royally."

"Yeah, right. You're the country boy who didn't know a business plan from your elbow a year ago and now this is all the gratitude you have?"

"For sure I'm grateful for you helping me pick up some business tips but lately they're more on how not to run a business – unless embezzlement, cocaine and bimbos are a success plan."

It was quiet for a second as Malone stared at Stephan with a look of intense hatred. His lower lip curled and he spat out the next words.

"Fuck you. You have no idea what you're talking about. And if you want to make allegations, then I'll see you in court."

"That's not a bad idea. You can show the judge the documents that spell out where all the government cash disappeared. We could all use a good laugh."

"And with your name down as president of one of the big entities, we'll be sharing a cell if that's what you want," Malone said raising his voice in anger.

Stephan kept calm. "I doubt it. I never signed anything and your forging my name on a federal check is all the proof I need to show your devious actions."

"Get the hell out of here." Malone waved an arm dismissively. "I'll get a release typed up when the secretary comes in and have her drop it off at the trailer by four. Leave your keys when you take your stuff from there."

"Don't worry, I'm already gone." Stephan tossed a key ring with a couple of keys on Malone's desk, turned and walked out through the outer office.

Malone called after him, "Hey, Mister Hot-shot, Tania wasn't that great in bed as she looked."

Stephan kicked a metal waste paper bin in front of him so it skidded across the floor crashing into the wall. He grabbed the first thing he could find on a neighboring desk, which was a telephone. Yanking the cable from the wall he threw the unit with all his might over the dividing wall of Malone's cubicle hoping for a direct hit.

Stephan was chilling with his Blem neighbors one night and got the latest update from Jack and Reedo whose musical activities had taken them into another universe while Stephan had been off exploring his own. He had been curious if the album his song was on had gotten any more airplay. They were sitting around in Stephan's living room enjoying some Elephant malt liquor and munching tortilla chips with a jar of salsa while Jack shared his favorite party story.

"Being new on the scene and playing a bunch of hot gigs got us a lot of outrageous party invites. Like you're not going to believe this – one night we had dinner with George at a restaurant off of La Cienega after going to a concert by Dr. John, the Night Tripper. Who shows up – The Doctor along with Alice Cooper! Next thing you know we're at the house of George's bandmate Ringo, somewhere above Sunset Boulevard."

"You're kidding me!" Stephan said grabbing for his beer.

Reedo added to the tale getting animated like he was

flailing his drumsticks at a gig. "It was crazy – when we waked in we saw the guys from Led Zeppelin surrounded by groupies and had to dodge David Crosby bouncing around looking for substances to abuse." Everyone laughed at the image of the space cowboy on patrol. "But what was so cool is that Michael bumped into his lifelong idol Peter Sellers waiting in line by the bathroom. He said he had been listening to our music courtesy of George and wanted to meet all of us. I got to watch the two of them swapping impressions of everything from Indian Rajas to French detectives for over an hour. I was laughing so hard I almost fell in the pool."

"And while all that was going on Tommy was trying to outdrink Rod Stewart," Jack said.

"Good luck," Stephan said.

"He gave up after he couldn't down any more rum and Cokes without passing out," Jack said laughing at the memory. "At the end of the evening when the crowd had thinned out, I had a long chat with Ringo who wanted to know all about me."

Reedo picked up the tale. "When we finally left the party, there was Sellers looking a bit lost because he couldn't find his limo driver. We gave him a lift in our van to someone's mansion in Beverly Hills."

The future was looking bright, until one day it was announced that George was moving to a different record company because of a deteriorating relationship with the current company's owners, mainly due to the record distribution being a disaster. Combined with this was a business review by his accountants, where he was advised to close his label, as the overall sales were not generating enough cash to make it a positive cash flow business. It was nothing personal, simply a practical business decision. The band had also suffered from the poor distribution from the parent company. While they had a good reception at the concerts and plenty of radio interviews during their thirty-city tour, they would go to store signings and there wouldn't be any records to sign.

Their album had started to get some more airplay and even the Fleetwood Mac bass player had noted that at some of the concerts the public had liked Jiva more than the Mac, the headliner. More support by the record company could have gotten their second single 'Take My Love' into the Top Ten, but as their business manager Alan was more a groupie of the rich and famous than a hard driving manager, the push to build on a successful launch didn't happen. The prophetic words of George when they were negotiating the original deal came back to haunt Jack, as once again it looked like Alan fumbled a golden opportunity.

Undaunted, Jiva was able to land at another label, Polydor Records, and get the go ahead for another album. Now they were back at square one, this time with a bigger company, which was both good and bad. The good part was the record company wouldn't be shutting down anytime soon, but the bad part was they were now one of many new bands on a huge roster. The competition for promotional funds was fierce, and as a fledgling group they had to prove themselves all over again.

The film world had been left behind so long ago that new

eager slaves occupied the regular production roles Stephan had toiled in earlier. After getting re-established back at Blem, Stephan only managed to find a couple of short-term jobs ranging from working with cartoon characters to helping a documentary filmmaker. The world of illusion had Stephan working side by side with Mickey and Goofy from Disneyland, putting together a multimedia show for the opening of a future city at their new Florida theme park.

While assembling 35mm slides at a studio in Hollywood, both cartoon characters were constantly arguing to see who would wear which costume at the Anaheim park the next day. Mickey was the most despised role because the mouse outfit attracted the more abusive children who got their laughs from kicking the creature's skinny legs. Whenever Stephan would escape the sweatshop environment and venture outside for fresh air, the lines of young male prostitutes along Santa Monica Boulevard doing their antics for cruising film executives would look at him like either competition or a customer.

Stephan's documentary experience took place on one of those cheerless foggy mornings that inspire suicides. His task was helping keep a cameraman from falling off a fishing boat while filming nets being reeled in bulging with a hefty catch. The newsreel image of piles of fish getting dumped on deck didn't materialize – only a few stray fish and discarded junk were caught in the nets. The low gray clouds that complemented the dawn chill emphasized the expedition's futility. While Stephan could keep his eye on the horizon and not get seasick, the cameraman experienced the opposite effect from trying to keep his eye to the camera's viewfinder. The poor fellow spent most of the day in the toilet, retching up his coffee and donuts from breakfast.

Finally, Stephan tried his hand working for a security company on projects managed by a couple of crazy British guys he met through the band. In spite of being in the country without a Green Card, their job was to pick up the illegal immigrants that arrived daily on Mexicano Airlines and baby-sit them in a hotel overnight before their deportation hearing the next morning. There was always a choice of exotic takeaway food to ease the boredom but sometimes that perk was offset by having to sprint down the street after a clever detainee who managed to wiggle out of the bathroom window. The immigration judge never thought to ask the snappy dressed pair with posh accents if their status was kosher.

The Brits set Stephan up in a guardhouse at the gate of a huge factory that manufactured respirator machines in the flatlands of an industrial zone between Venice and the airport. Stephan worked the graveyard shift and would have to answer alarm calls like when the electronic map would indicate a door was disturbed at the most desolate area of the complex facing an endless rail yard fronting an open field. Walking through the huge factory wired to the max on industrial strength coffee and paranoid from smoking some grass, he would have his .457 Magnum with hollow-point bullets drawn as he edged through the massive complex. There were all kinds of whirring machines and the ominous sound of breathing coming from every corner where respirators were being tested like one hundred Darth

Vaders hissing at him. He jumped at every sound wanting to shoot anything that moved. Needless to say, the late hours and nerve-wracking tension of false alarms in dangerous locations combined with terminal boredom soon ended the arrangement.

After these short episodes, the opportunities dwindled, and in spite of an offer to work as an extra in a porn film, Stephan started to contemplate more serious options. Although Mac was asking for more help on his screenplay, Stephan needed cash now, not in some unknown future, which made him open to any and all possibilities. He visited some job agencies to find publishing-related work and landed a temporary assignment at Playboy Publications. He would be working at their headquarters, located in a tall office building adorned with their trademark happy-face rabbit, at the end of Sunset Boulevard's commercial area.

Instead of the bachelor dream of hallways full of models in skimpy bunny costumes, the gay editor Stephan assisted was harassing him with cute pats on the ass. The job didn't last too long, and while the job agency tried to find him further work Stephan put in more time on his book project, in hopes of getting a first draft completed that he could begin to show around to editors and agents.

The Blem Mafia's extended family included a small house halfway down the block that usually had a VW bus stuffed with surfboards parked in the front yard. It complemented a custom Ford low-rider pickup the Mexican neighbors across the street showcased in their garden, in place of an ornate birdbath or plastic pink flamingos.

The low-slung house with faded paint was home to a surfer dude, his beach babe business partner plus a natural living freak that worked for an organic ice cream company as well as a Venezuelan lady who made pottery. Will was a blond-haired surfer who was usually hanging in Hermosa or Redondo Beach at a health food restaurant between sets of big waves. To finance his lifestyle, he regularly drove motor homes back and forth from Mexico with his roommate and partner named Brandi, along with an old retired couple they hired for the occasion.

Their cover as a family returning from vacation deflected any inquiries at the border that might lead to discovering the kilos of grass stuffed into every possible free space. Will handled his business discretely to avoid raising questions from the landlord or straight neighbors. Maybe the expensive Persian rugs in his bedroom would have been a clue and a thin cover story of being a rug importer was the excuse for his income. Big on health food and carrot juice, he would be grinding away with his juicer every day, working his way through a fifty-pound bag of carrots, drinking so much at times that his skin would turn orange.

When Stephan would spot the van out front, he would bang on the door to get a dose of liquid energy from Will. One day they were toasting life with carrot juice flavored with fresh ginger, while washing down some organic corn chips. They were sitting on the back deck of the house under the bougainvillea philosophizing, while another smog-enhanced sunset colored the high clouds.

"Dude, you should take up surfing. Put that asana stuff

to good use," Will said, swilling a large gulp from his juice that left orange foam on his moustache. "Get you close to nature. Yeah, find that balance."

"I'm going to surprise you once and show up at one of your sessions," Stephan answered reaching for some chips.

"Cool. Some days when you're waiting for a good set there's this sense of timelessness and detachment because the waves will come when they come. No sooner, no later."

"That's how life is in India. Later can mean anything from two hours to the next day. That's when you start to see the now is all you have."

"Right on. It's like those soul surfers who say they go into the Zen on a big wave because you gotta be in the moment riding a ton of water or you're fish food. Want another libation, bro?"

"I'm fine, thanks. Where's Brandi? I didn't see her airbrushing in the garage today."

"She's off somewhere, probably down at the beach selling T-shirts."

Brandi was a perpetually tanned, petite blond who created tropical T-shirts between Mexican vacations. She was constantly in motion and drove a small Honda like it was a Grand Prix racecar. A spoiled rich girl whose daddy owned a major car repair chain, she epitomized the California blond stereotype. Life had been a lark and visits to Mexico broke the monotony of ski trips to Argentina when it was off-season in Switzerland.

"I liked the modeling session last week when she had her sister and those other honeys showing off the shirts," Stephan said.

"Totally, dude. That tall brunette was like, bodacious. Sure you don't want some wheatgrass juice?"

"I'm cool."

"Me and Bruce are trying to elevate our diets. He swears we can be bretharians if we stick to the raw foods. Elevating ourselves up the food chain to be able to eventually live off light and breath."

"I heard. But Bruce puts alfalfa sprouts on everything from his avocado sandwiches to the morning granola."

"The guy is a bit extreme. He's a legend among the jungle bunny naturopaths around Santa Barbara because he was caught with a trunk full of stolen avocados. Earned him a GTA title – Grand Theft Avocado."

"I don't want to imagine him eating the left-over fudge ripple ice-cream he delivers with sprouts on top," Stephan said.

"Right on. Bruce wants to move to the eastern side of the Andes because they're the steepest mountains in the world. They act as a shield as the earth rotates so airborne debris passes over the base. The ultimate pollution-free environment."

"I wish him luck dodging the pygmy head-hunters and fifty-foot pythons. I'll stick around here and take my chances. That famous nutritionist who developed a fruitarian diet died when he got hit by a truck crossing the street, so right eating didn't extend his life any."

A couple of weeks later Stephan was banging on the surfer's door, as he hadn't seen the bus out front for many days. The curtains were all drawn and after a short wait the door quietly opened. Jennifer, the pottery artist watched him for a second through the screen door before she invited him in. They sat in the patio where she was painting the glaze on some South-American-inspired red clay pots. Her long curly black hair was tied back in a ponytail so her round friendly face was nicely framed. She was wearing cut-offs and a bright red halter top.

She explained the cause of the secrecy. "The conductors noticed Will when he was riding the train back from Arizona last week with a huge steamer trunk full of grass. The trunk was confiscated from the baggage compartment before he got to Union Station."

"Will wouldn't be hard to notice. Nobody under retirement age rides trains these days, so a longhaired blond dude in a Hawaiian shirt had to stand out."

"Will sneaked into the baggage room in the station while the clerks were off trying to locate the police. He got away in a taxi but the police knew his address from the baggage label. For the past week a phone company truck has been parked in front of the house," Jennifer said.

"I wondered what that was all about. I thought maybe one of the neighbors worked for the phone company and had borrowed it."

Will never came home so Jennifer ended up shipping his possessions to his new home in Miami. Bruce disappeared, afraid that with his GTA conviction he could get in trouble and Brandi decided the snow was about right in the Swiss Alps. Jennifer was the only one left and wasn't sure if she would attempt to keep the house with some new roommates or also move out.

"This is indeed a sad day for wave riders and artists," Stephan said.

The band had been bummed at the news because the free samples, both legal and illegal, disappeared and the family dynamic was broken. Reedo and Jack had been frequent guests, as well as Stephan and Maceo, mostly because of Jennifer and Brandi and their girlfriends who hung around and modeled T-shirts. Maceo had become addicted to the organic cappuccino ice-cream that he ate for breakfast provided from the loose cartons Bruce scavenged from the delivery truck he drove.

Not long after the train incident, Stephan had moved out to the desert and when he returned, the house had been taken over by some students that included yet another natural living colleague named Stu Stickler. The crew called him Dr. Voodoo because he was an acupuncture student, practicing on whoever would sit still long enough.

Shortly after Stephan's return from the desert he was surprised when Will appeared one morning at the door of his bungalow.

"Dude! What's going on?" came the greeting from a familiar face hidden behind huge aviator sunglasses and a Miami Dolphins baseball cap.

"My man, whassup?" Stephan said. They slapped hands and Will quickly stepped in and made himself at home in the living room, flopping down on the sofa. Stephan commented, "I thought you had disappeared off the planet after your adventure."

"Let's just say the LAPD accelerated my plans to move

on. Miami is so cool with all the crazy Cubans running around and the water is this amazing blue. Man, you got to come and check it out."

"Sounds good to me. I got the story from Jennifer about your last escapade in these parts. You're not worried being back in town?" Stephan sat on his desk chair, leaning back and putting his elbows on the edge of the desk.

"No way. The cops have too much other shit to worry about, and besides with no evidence, they have no case," Will said.

"Excellent."

"But I decided to stay in Florida and operate my business from there. I've been working with a dude I know here in LA who is my local contact. I ship him half a bale every couple of weeks and he makes the rounds to customers."

"You ship the stuff?"

"Yeah, dig this. The federal government is my partner. I send it as auto parts via Express Overnight Mail and because it's internal mail inside the good ol' U.S. of A. the customs people don't check the shit." They both laughed at the absurdity of the scenario.

"That's fucking amazing."

"It's like we used to talk – the whole world is an illusion and if you believe something's real, then it is. And if you want the public to think you're shipping auto parts they believe you. I pick up the bales down at the docks right off of the banana boats." Will was stretched out on the sofa with his flip-flops falling off his tanned feet as he extended his legs.

"Sounds better than motor homes," Stephan said.

"For sure. TJ is starting to get hot with narcs crawling over any vehicles that look even remotely suspicious trying to cross the border."

"That Operation Intercept Nixon set up along the border back in '69 was the feds' genius idea for solving the drug problem."

"It was just PR, man. There's more shit than ever coming into the country," Bill said proudly.

"Demand drives supply."

"I heard you had a falling-out with Malone and are looking for some income."

They briefly discussed the dissolution of Stephan's relationship with Malone and Great Impressions Publishing.

"How would you like to help me out for a few weeks and make some quick cash?"

"You mean like a train ride from Arizona?" Stephan asked smiling.

"Nothing so obvious. My man here in town is taking off for six or eight weeks on a little vacation cruise and I need someone to cover for him. All you gotta do is pick up a package at the post office every couple of weeks and distribute the contents to a few guys around LA. We're talking ten grand a month, cash, for close to two months' work."

"You're kidding."

"Seriously. Each half a bale weighs fifty pounds; you make a hundred off each pound. Boom, five grand," Will said.

It was a tempting offer. Stephan would have time to work on his book and still be able to clear out some debts like the car he bought on a payment plan and credit card charges from when money didn't seem to be an issue. "Sounds great. But going to jail would be a real drag."

"Don't worry about that. There's enough cash put aside to bail you out and handle any legal expenses if need be. This operation has been running for years without a single problem."

"Would I have to smoke myself silly to do quality control or what?"

"I buy only the best Colombian gold. And if you promise to keep a secret, I'll tell you how I check the potency," Will said leaning forward confidentially.

"Okay."

"I chew a little sample and from that I can tell how strong it is. If my customers knew I didn't smoke it, they would doubt my judgment, but nobody's complained until now." Sensing Stephan's hesitation Will said, "Look, I know you have your values and focus on pure living, and I respect that, so why don't you take some time to think about it? If it's not for you, that's cool, I have some other people I can talk to. I just need to move on this soon as my guy is leaving town in a few days."

"When do you need an answer?"

"How about we meet this afternoon around four at that falafel stand in Venice?"

"Sounds good."

Will adjusted the baseball cap low on his forehead and from the door said, "Hasta la vista, dude."

Stephan initially had his doubts, as his attempt to lead

a healthy lifestyle made him avoid too many intoxicants other than the occasional beer, lest they dull his experience and the temptation to indulge would be ever-present. One of his first thoughts was how he'd clearly given Greg the message that he wasn't supporting his shadowy lifestyle. So now if Stephan were to deal drugs, then he'd be betraying his own beliefs. He could only imagine what Greg would say – some smart-assed remark with a smirk on his face. Then again, he didn't necessarily have to let Greg know what he was up to. Still, Stephan was in conflict. Ten grand a month... imagine how well he could live on that. And then he thought of Greg's free and easy ways, and how open Greg was. Maybe a more bohemian way of life could also loosen up Stephan's straight existence that was almost too rigid at times with the desire to always do the right thing, and follow the latest sets of golden rules be they Buddhist or Christian.

He also thought back on some of the conversations he had with Lila where she also accused him of being too mentally stiff, with his fixed beliefs and conceptual approach to life. Stephan considered the offer from all sides and with the lack of other options to find income, combined with his pressing financial needs, the proposition finally didn't sound too bad. It was only for a few weeks, so he might as well take the opportunity while it was there. He didn't know when he would find a decent job but this could provide a cushion to cover his needs until something real came along. Ignoring any possible negative consequences, he decided to say yes. They agreed on terms and Will gave Stephan his associate's name to contact for the customer list and to get the necessary client introductions made.

Stephan was nervous as hell the first time he had to pick up a shipment. He had to wait in line at the main post office in Santa Monica, wondering if the package had broken open or been somehow compromised, meaning a one-way ticket to the county jail the locals called the Crossbar Hotel, providing three hots and a cot. The lady at the counter took the receipt Stephan had received in the mail and scrutinized it closely. She spoke to a colleague in the back room and returned to the window. Stephan had almost left at that point, afraid of being busted, but he held his nerve with a couple of deep breaths that rolled up from his lower belly to the top of his lungs and back down again.

The clerk said he had to go around to the loading dock in the back of the building. Relieved, he retrieved his car and parked in the loading zone, finding a three-foot square package weighing fifty pounds waiting on the edge of the loading platform, labeled auto parts, with a fake Miami garage as the shipper. It barely fit into the back of his Japanese hatchback. The contents were half a bale of grass; Colombian gold that smelled of mountain earth and verdant jungle.

The triple beam scale Stephan was meant to borrow was being recalibrated after an accidental tumble, so he visited the current distributor who could help him get started with his packaging. Ricardo was one of those characters who were sure it was still 1967 even though it was ten years later. He not only dressed the part, starting with a ponytail halfway down his back, but made sure his lifestyle was as anti-establishment as they come. But appearances could be deceiving and while this time-warped individual was a monument to the counterculture ideal, there was one minor twist – Ricardo worked at the Jet Propulsion Laboratory in Pasadena, so was in fact a rocket scientist. The research labs, even those doing government defense work, were used to all manner of eccentrics, so when Ricardo would rumble into the parking lot on his chopped Harley and stride into the office wearing not much more than a denim vest, leather pants and ass-kicker boots, nobody batted an eye. He had helped land a man on the moon, so who cares what you did on your weekends.

Ricardo's girlfriend was a jeweler in Venice, so Stephan arranged to meet him at her small studio a half a block up from the beach in a trashed-out alley. The lady was showing off a recent pendant she had cast out of silver – an exact miniature of an erect penis. Ricardo proudly explained that he had been the model. Ricardo took Stephan to a Safeway supermarket just above Wilshire, at around six, when most people were home having dinner. They had taken along large clumps of grass they had broken off the bale, packed loosely in brown paper shopping bags. They went into a backroom where Ricardo's friend the produce manager set them up in a quiet corner where they weighed the grass into one-pound units. Stephan was almost too paranoid to speak, expecting a manager or bag boy to burst in upon their activity. Ricardo nonchalantly dropped handfuls of grass into large zip-lock Baggies. The bright-eyed dealer explained that's how it worked in this business – by being so obvious about something, nobody would even think twice about what you were up to. The public generally gave the benefit of the doubt to an individual's integrity.

Stephan tried to balance his changing lifestyle of nights visiting customers and sampling the product with some morning meditation and yoga classes. Word got around about his business and he was getting party invites from all kinds of people who knew he would be generous with his materials. Stephan's sensibilities were slowly getting lost in the swirl of the permanent Bogotá smog. Acknowledging the warning flags of a questionable business in the desert should have made him wiser to the perils of a new venture. The clues were all there for any rational human to see. And in the end Stephan felt alone – he couldn't be sure of his friends' motivations to want to see him and he learned slowly that he couldn't trust his customers. Not even the police were a welcome sight. This meant it was about karma and good vibes, trusting in a benevolent universe. In other words, he was more of a fool than any of the deluded seekers of fame and fortune he shared the freeways and bars with. And the law of the jungle was the rule, as customers ranging from gang suppliers in the middle of South Central to the Lebanese mafia and Venice beach bums, who would each find a way to test Stephan's relative innocence.

Deals were done in shopping center parking lots (the rule of something too obvious to be suspicious worked well in these situations), by local parks in the quiet suburbs or any number of funky, low-rent apartments from Hollywood to Redondo Beach with indifferent neighbors. On one trip the police stopped him for rolling through a crosswalk in the black ghetto when someone was just stepping onto it from the curb. He was let go with a warning to be more respectful; the police probably didn't want any incidents that would trigger a riot. The sports bag on the backseat remained untouched while Stephan's heart was pounding loud enough to drown out the radio.

Maybe driving to the middle of the black ghetto at two in the morning with a sports sack full of drugs, and a return trip with thousands of dollars in cash would have been an indicator that common sense had been forgotten. It was all about being cool, but then how cool can you be as the only white person in a five-mile radius, with no protection other than the customer you were delivering to, who was affiliated with so many black gangs that even the UN was an amateur organization by comparison.

19

IF YOU WRITE IT, THEY WILL COME

The writing dragged on and progress was slow but Stephan's novel acted as a balance to his illegal activities. And if the publishing business had been a time robber, then working as Miami Will's driver also had its detracting effects with late nights of partying being the prime cause of delays. And while the original story of Rama was a two thousand-page epic that made Stephan's condensation of it a major undertaking, the creative process was its own reward, touching him somewhere deeper than the temporary flashes of pleasure he got from the product he was distributing.

The act of creation gave him a sense of control over his future, the fulfillment of bringing a vision to life and a way of adding to the turning of the great wheel, to help the planet move from the kaliyuga age of darkness to the satyuga, the age of truth. But nagging doubts about the validity of his efforts challenged the warm glow of his bodhisattva dream of Buddhist compassion, and he would occasionally ask himself if in the end anyone would want to read it.

Even with a project to anchor him, there were times Stephan still felt unfulfilled. Part of it was due to the nature of pursuing a higher experience that required constant inspiration, as inner peace surely existed but its nature wasn't self-reminding. The sources of inspiration grew thin and were easily lost with shortcuts taking the place of effort. Not realizing the full potential of the publishing business he had been building, while having been at the edge of success, was annoying whenever he remembered the situation.

Also, the pull of recognition and accomplishment was slowly compelling and addictive in a town where nothing else mattered. More simply, the Hollywood bug had bitten Stephan and he was starting to itch. Partying with film people customers had made him feel part of the lifestyle for fleeting instances and made him want to belong. Helping feed this feverish mania that at some time or another seized even the most stouthearted citizen was Maceo. While Mac moonlighted as an airline's reservations voice on an 800 number by day, in the evening he worked without stop on his scripts. Like their neighbor across the driveway who endlessly applied paint to canvas, with canvasses stacked three deep against every wall, the same single-minded purpose led to a bungalow stacked to the rafters with piles of script drafts, 'how to write a script' books and endless reference texts from which to cull ideas, information and inspiration.

Stephan's flexibility of schedule gave him a lot of free time as his 'job' of delivery boy meant about four of five drives every week, as each delivery provided sufficient material for the customer to do their local distribution for many days. This then left Stephan with plenty of time for hanging out in Venice on skates and barhopping between the outdoor cafés in one endless happy hour. But in spite of the free and easy times there was a sense of a lack of purpose nagging at him and while his writing project was the main driver he justified his frequent inactivity as a form of writer's block and by considering this lifestyle as research. How could he write about a noble person slumming with his chin up if he didn't live some experience of that himself?

Eventually Mac engaged Stephan to help edit his latest project for a share of potential profits. Sensing a quicker payday than his work in progress and an alternative income to his soon-to-expire delivery job, Stephan jumped at the chance. Mac had a couple of projects going and during the frequent visits from his neighbor, bounced ideas off Stephan. Mac's latest script was part political thriller with some humanitarian elements based on the Founding Fathers' words and actions. There was also some Native American imagery thrown in for good measure, in the form of a twentieth century Pocahontas, spouting traditional wisdom.

Stephan succumbed to the success bug and figured he could network through his range of contacts to sell this script – all it took was someone who knew someone. It would be easy with an idea this hot to get an actor with sensitivity interested. Someone like Robert Redford or Clint Eastwood would be perfect in the role of a pilot turned astronaut running for president. The role would request someone who could express the courage of a man who believed in the spiritual values of the Founding Fathers, articulating them with a statesman-like quality and at the same time being able to commune with Native Americans, passing a peace pipe around a ceremonial fire.

Mac was convinced he had the ultimate script that tied in the recent presidential election and bicentennial celebrations. It was also an expression of his accumulated knowledge of mystical arcana in the form of America's obscure symbols, like the pyramid with radiant eye, eagles with thirteen tail feathers and George Washington's wooden teeth.

Fuelled by coffee and donuts in some marathon discussion sessions, the script started to take shape. They were racing the clock because given a year's typical production time and related business it meant that for it to be released within the memory of the recent 1976 two-hundred-year birthday of America, they had to hustle the script now, pitching the idea wherever an opportunity presented itself. There was also research required to flesh out the idea and a need to find allies to champion the vision and ideally slip the writer some money so Mac could take time off to write and rewrite.

Mac and Stephan tossed ideas back and forth and reshaped the structure every time a new plot twist seemed key to progressing the story. They bantered dialogue, taking turns of putting themselves into each character to get the conversation flow sounding real. The nights got late and after weeks of Mac's rewrites, they rewarded themselves with a six-pack of Dos Equis when the latest draft looked presentable.

Stephan plucked up his courage knowing the odds were seriously stacked against him and had taken to flogging the story during the day to anyone he could find. He started with the TV screenwriter that worked next to the old publishing offices in Producers Studio. The writer had a few kind words of encouragement but had become cynical from his own lack of success. He was still looking to sell his second TV script, so he could only wish them good luck before asking what Stephan thought the Dodgers chances of winning the World Series were.

Stephan tried everyone he knew at the production companies he had worked for and all the publishing connections; just in case somebody had a link to a person of influence. But like all the dealmakers in Hollywood, the execs were constantly getting hit with ideas left and right. Every single person – waiter, waitress, bag boy at Ralph's and the guy cleaning the pool was an aspiring actor or actress from Des Moines, Iowa and the rest wanted to be screenwriters. Thank the director Spielberg for his film *Jaws*, the surprise summer blockbuster about a giant fish terrorizing a small coastal town – big concepts got attention nowadays. After all, that was 'shark on beach' and Mac and Stephan's was: 'young president fights off evil corporation to return America to its true values' (think JFK).

Stephan got some honest feedback from his first boss in the film business, Bill, who graciously spared ten minutes to hear the pitch. It was not his specialty as he had moved onto romantic comedies. However, if it could be rewritten to be a humorous story with a down-to-earth hero and an airhead bimbo they could talk.

After many false starts and dried-up leads, Stephan's marketing enthusiasm was beginning to wane. He started to sound like yet another enthusiastic guy with a story – not much different than the waiter at Pizza Hut who had taken a weekend script-writing workshop. When Stephan almost started to believe the uselessness of his efforts, but too proud to admit it to Mac, it was like a miracle when Lila stepped in and offered her help. It was conditional, as all deals in this city turn out to be. In exchange for getting the script into production, she wanted to play the Indian girl. Even though they had discussed the project when they first met, it had been forgotten as they had drifted their separate ways, but now they were both at a point of readiness in their respective careers.

Stephan hadn't been seeing too much of Lila except at yoga class (where he had also been trolling for sponsors), because while he was in the desert she had been shacking up with the British director who had given her a minor role in his latest production. He had left for England after completion and Lila was back at her home, but they seemed to have both been satisfied with their temporary oh-so-typical Hollywood arrangement. Now the frequency of her meetings with Stephan increased as Lila, with all her ambition, was starting to feel like she was selling out her soul to get ahead. She confided in Stephan that she was more drawn to a life of higher pursuits, and as a result was spending more time at Bilkem's getting enough hours (and paying enough money) to finish off being certified as a yoga teacher.

Lila, with her dedication to making it in the film industry, was getting used to men going after her body. It was not only the relentless pawing of Bilkem under the guise of subtle corrections that trained her to be non-attached to the shell of the soul. Trying to get a job in this city also requested that an actress be able to use her many talents to her advantage to beat out the competition. While she really liked Stephan, he didn't have the horsepower to get her into a film. An internal debate she had been having since they first met continued with their burgeoning friendship that weighed the value of letting go to her feelings and free-falling into the blissful state of love or else holding back and having a companion that could serve as escort and surrogate partner to satisfy that basic social need.

Some days Lila would tell Stephan to bring his coolest Armani bought with his illegal proceeds along to yoga class so he could escort her to a private screening at a studio after the workout. Only lack of cleavage was as career devastating as not having a good-looking man to escort you. If you looked like a real loser who couldn't even land a guy to go out with, how could you be expected to carry a role on the screen? But even though Stephan was asked to be her escort, Lila would discretely leave the class early so one and all would know she had an important appointment, because a lot of industry heavyweights were always in and out of the class. Somehow it seemed to Stephan she was articulating through her actions the unspoken emotions she really felt but didn't have the courage to say out loud. He played along in hopes maybe she would finally see through her limitations. After Tania, Stephan's sense of what a relationship could be had taken a more serious note. He knew that Lila had the potential to be a caring and true companion if she could see through her insecurity about not being successful and let it unfold with the base of a good partner to support her.

Lila worked the crowd at the latest screening in a small theater on a studio lot while Stephan stood around awkwardly by the drinks table not knowing any of the people but ever hopeful to pitch his script to anyone who stood still long enough. Lila was giving orders to her agent who could only nod in agreement at the brassy delivery and even telling, not asking, a director to call her for a screen test for his next film. Later, when walking Lila to her car she clung to Stephan like a lost little girl who had just wandered out of a party for grown-ups.

After the evening of the screening, Stephan had a quiet dinner with Lila at her small house in a respectable part of Venice, as far inland as one could be before the LA city limits. She was back to acting normal again; not having an audience she could behave like his tomboy sister. It was almost like she was testing the waters of what a relationship would be like, without having to make a commitment. And Stephan, the ever-hopeful bachelor looking for love, could make himself available in the event things would finally move to another level as they both new subconsciously was their eventual destiny.

Lila could flirt, tease, and in the case of a director or hot producer have a little physical contact if it kept her in the producer's mind when it came to casting time. It was just another business transaction, as there were no emotions involved. But somewhere her soul knew otherwise, and Stephan was her anchor to the deeper side of yoga that the Hindu gymnastics that Bilkem pushed everyone through didn't touch. They both knew they liked each other and had a mutual physical attraction and for some reason the spark never turned to a flame. Stephan wondered if she resisted giving into her obvious feelings because she hadn't yet landed an A-list actor or Oscar winning director for a partner and resulting benefits. He also suspected a bit of mother-daughter competition that drove her to show she could be as successful in the film industry as her mother had been. Once she had proved this to herself she could then do what she pleased without any feeling of inadequacy. He had hoped her yoga studies would help her understand it was all about the journey, not the destination. It was obvious that Lila was selectively promiscuous but for her to get together with him was a serious matter, not a one-night stand to land a role. He waited and made himself available as best as he could, hoping one day what was apparent to him as a perfect match would also become apparent to her.

What Stephan didn't see was that by thinking too much he had missed the hidden message. It wasn't only about having any guy friend to go out with but in fact hanging around together and taking him to screenings was Lila's roundabout way of getting to know him better in a social situation to validate he could be a partner publicly as well as in bed. As Lila was slowly opening up to him, Stephan missed the obvious signs as his thoughts still drifted back to his desert encounter, distracting him from what was slowly unfolding in front of his eyes.

Lila knew just the producer to pitch the script to. Never mind that he had shamelessly dry humped her against the antique French Louis XIV armoire in his office on the last visit, after he consumed a couple of shots of tequila, a Quaalude and a dozen lines of coke; he had the power to green light projects. Always juggling scripts and multiple development deals, Bob Sampson was a rock star Hollywood producer as flamboyant as anyone would hope to find, who had made enough 'fuck you' money to tell the world to go screw itself while he chose the projects he wanted to make.

He was as hot as the noonday sun at the equator from a low-budget flick called *Video Girls* with a good-girl-beats-the-odds theme and Top Ten songs in the background. The film earned more than eight times its cost, with an equally successful soundtrack album. It was like picking the winning horse at the Hollywood Park racetrack with hundred-to-one odds. As a result, the studio had enough faith in his ability to spot a winning story, guide it through to filming and onto the screen that they were willing to put up development money if the pitch was good enough. His next project was about the daredevil exploits of a highflying Air Force bad boy called *Cockpit Hero*, and had all the promise of another mega blockbuster. Lila felt confident that she could sell the story Stephan and Mac had spun in their late-night work sessions to Bob with sincerity and passion. For the killer pitch that would also land her in the role of the female lead she would use the sofa next time, as the armoire left her pulling 17th century splinters out of her well-shaped behind.

Lila got on his agenda, made the pitch with a five-page treatment and received a favorable reaction. It was another typical meeting where Bob managed to down a couple of tumblers of Scotch, and inhale a half a gram of coke while Lila, without knowing it, came within inches of having her anus lose its virginity while they romped on his leather sofa.

At the last second, Bob either slipped, was too loaded or maybe just complacent, wanting to save some energy for the black lady with the whip that was visiting his Beverly Hills mansion later, so aiming too low, shot his load across Lila's breasts instead. With his head close to hers, she caught a whiff of a scent she knew well – Preparation H. Sampson was using the hemorrhoid cream like others who believed it would temporarily tighten the wrinkles on their worn-out face. After satisfactorily consummating a verbal agreement that would put Lila in the title role of the Indian lady, Bob agreed to take a meeting with the story development team.

The meeting with Stephan and Mac was at a nondescript coffee shop not far from Bob's studio offices in North Hollywood. Bob was dressed from head to toe in black, starting with a French T-shirt that probably cost as much as Stephan and Mac's combined wardrobe, silk Italian slacks with black crocodile skin belt and Gucci loafers without socks. It was clear whom the illegally parked Turbo Carrera Porsche out front with metallic black paint belonged to.

Mac had a 120-page script with him that he lay on the table to show it wasn't just talk, but that he had a real product. The title, Union of the State, was printed on a cover page in red, white and blue letters.

"So, what's the opening again?" Bob hadn't read too much of the treatment, evidently relying on Lila's summary, kicking back in the booth waiting for the pitch.

Mac started in seriously like a scholar delivering his doctorate dissertation with an upright posture adding to the effect. "A former astronaut is running for president and wants to bring back the original values of the Founding Fathers and help the Native American cause. His girlfriend is an Indian."

"Yeah and then?" Bob said in a bored voice as he leaned forward and put his arms on the table while looking for a waitress.

"There are some big corporations who don't like his back-to-nature philosophy and want to sabotage his plans, because they really want the Indian land for the oil," Mac said not quite indignantly but with a light tone of that it should have been obvious. Stephan watched the conversation waiting for an opening as he held his coffee cup in both hands like a monk in a tea ceremony.

"Now we're getting somewhere. Let's go back to the opening. You say he's an astronaut – how about he's also an adventurer and wants to test a rocket car on the Bonneville Salt Flats. Set the new land speed record blasting around in this big jet car, with some booming patriotic soundtrack to inspire everyone." Bob sat back against the padded booth.

"We were thinking more about the inspiration coming from the forgotten words of the Founding Fathers," Stephan said looking intently at Bob trying to steer the discussion to the real meaning behind the images.

"I dig what you're saying, but forget that shit. That's okay for a history class. We want people to watch this movie and get emotionally involved. If people want to read the Declaration of Independence, they can go to a library. The public want to be entertained," Bob said as he leaned forward stirring a big spoon of sugar into the coffee the waitress delivered from his hand signal.

"I'm not sure," Stephan said. He pushed himself back from the table to emphasize his point while Mac had a look that said he wasn't sure whether to retrieve the script or dive in again.

"Look, I've made some monster movies and my gut feel says go with the hero story. What's the deal with the Indian chick?" Bob was getting interested again.

"She's a teacher who is trying to get her people educated and off the reservation," Mac said trying to add an edge of excitement to his voice.

"Good, sounds like a start. How about she gets kidnapped by the corporation and used to keep the race car guy from running for office."

"We didn't agree he's a driver," Stephan said missing the point of Bob's attempt to bridge the differences.

"And I didn't agree to help you either, if I don't like the story. Look, you've got nothing more than a half-baked idea. I'm trying to help 'cause I think there may be something here." Bob was trying to sound like he was appreciative of good story telling, someone with culture.

"Okay, we'll think about it." Mac was starting to sound like he wanted out. "We thought of her more like Jimmy Carter's wife, supporting him on his presidential campaign," Mac said again with a precise tone as if it were a history class. He tentatively touched the edge of the script as if to take it back and show it to someone else.

"Ain't gonna work. We need some drama and some excitement and need a babe. Not a dumpy middle-aged housewife who's married to a peanut farmer from Georgia, if you know what I mean. Then how about the corporation hires a hit-man to sabotage the astronaut's car when he's doing a test drive?"

"The guy's a retired spaceman, not a daredevil," Mac said.

"Nope, gotta have some jazzy stuff to keep it moving," Bob said like he was lecturing a class on film studies and sitting up straight he continued. "Let me explain my philosophy to you. The public wants to be entertained not lectured about history or anything else. You gotta start big to get their interest with a blockbuster opening. Something like a fiery explosion of some kind or a spectacular crash with cars tumbling like dominoes. Then you have to show how the hero is vulnerable, by beating him down into the dust. Then by his own hard efforts he's able to raise himself out of the rut he's been tossed into. By the end of the film he's made a comeback – the loser guy who triumphs over all the obstacles that keep piling up that make it look impossible to get what he's after. Then you got to add some cool music for a soundtrack. I like the Indian thing. Could have Indian dancing girls in leather outfits, sweating around a fire with primitive drumming punched up with some synthesizers." The loser guy who triumphs was the story of Sampson's childhood that Lila had explained to Stephan after hearing it on every visit to Bob's office.

Stephan played the diplomat as he could see Mac ready to leave the meeting out of pride. "What you're saying isn't impossible; it's another way of telling the story." Mac continued to look blank. "How about we see what we can do with some of your input and come up with a second draft?"

Bob agreed and asked some questions about the characters' motivation and asked if they couldn't build in some fancy-dress ball or similar scene with fashionably dressed people. Mac broke his silence and tried to explain that the story wasn't an action movie, but one with meaning and insight. Bob assured him that public taste was more in favor of a simple plot in black and white, with a lot of dramatic moments, something he kept referring to as 'big concept'. He believed the auteur theory from French cinema of the director as God should be revised with the producer as the ultimate driver of a film's vision, with him as the lead proponent.

"We'll work on it," was the reply from Mac. Sampson carried on. Next, he wanted the hero and the Indian girl to have a romantic involvement by mid-story to set up a dramatic ending with gallant rescue. Some kind of scene with a tumble in a sweat lodge, where their sexual encounter could be tastefully filmed through the haze of the steam was important. It would make a soft edge to the action that would follow. Naturally it would be performed to the rhythmic beat of native drums on top of a disco soundtrack. They might even think about a tribute to the classic Westerns, with a cowboy-versus-Indian segment, where a platoon of jeeps led by the hero rescues the Indian girl from a stampede of renegade, but noble savages with war paint and Winchester rifles.

At the end of the whirlwind discussion, the script owners' heads were buzzing from the speed and intensity of the story conference and the three or four cups of coffee they each consumed to keep up with Bob. His motormouth dissertation had only been interrupted by a couple of trips to the bathroom, where he would return with the telltale couple of strong sniffs to further inhale any loose flakes of coke that were stuck to his nasal passage. A grungy gold Tinkerbelle fairy pendant on a thick gold rope chain hung outside his shirt with the fairy's tail clearly shaped into a miniature spoon.

They talked about the development route and Bob said he was convinced they were onto something, and he could help them get a deal. If they could make the changes he suggested, he would pitch it to the contacts he had at the studio and get Mac some up-front money to complete the script. Stephan and Mac could barely hide their elation, as they were as close to getting a movie made as anyone could in this unforgiving town. Never mind it wasn't their original concept, better a deal in production than a script in the closet.

Bob quickly glanced at his heavy gold Rolex and excused himself because of another meeting, followed by a definitive, "It's a wrap."

On the way out, crossing the parking lot, Bob casually asked if the guys had any smoke. Stephan was eager to please and said he could help in a show of bravado to indicate he wasn't a lightweight, but also a player with some horsepower. Everyone in town was looking for primo grass and uncut coke, so any new contact was an edge. Boys and their toys – if you had good drugs, you had respect.

"What you got?" Bob asked.

Stephan pulled a bomber out of his shirt pocket, lit it, and passing it over, said it was a sample, adding, "How much do you need – quarter, half, kilo?”

“You got a quarter pound of something decent?” Sampson said through a constricted voice holding in the smoke.

“Colombian gold, fresh off the boat.”

“Cool. How much you get for a pound?”

“Five hundred is the going rate,” Stephan said.

“No problemo.”

Stephan had four ounces in the trunk of his car bagged for a late-afternoon delivery, but could swing by Blem to replace it for the customer. Stephan handed a brown paper bag to Bob and said, “Enjoy.”

Bob stuffed the paper sack in his satchel, pulled out his wallet extracting the cash and handed it to Stephan. He walked off puffing on the joint that he hadn’t passed back to share with the two guys, as he fired up his Porsche. Before he slipped into the traffic, Bob yelled out, “So get your butts in gear and let’s make us a movie.”

After not seeing each other for what seemed a lifetime, Jack was explaining to Stephan the dynamics of the rock business with existential detachment over pizza and beer. “The tour went well and put the band on the top of the charts with gold and multiple platinum records to hang on the wall. We’re talking about sales in the double-digit millions with a number one album, which translates into Ferraris, private jets, Malibu beach houses.” Stephan stopped eating and looked at Jack in disbelief. Jack continued, “But unfortunately, it was Fleetwood Mac not Jiva, raking in the royalty checks from being million sellers.”

"That blows my mind. It could have just as easily been Jiva," Stephan said shaking his head. "Fame is such a fickle mistress. It's like two people standing next to each other on stage and one is in the spotlight while the other is invisible. You can be in the right place, at the right time and by chance miss the glory," Stephan said.

"Sure wish I was able to operate the lighting on this story. Getting stuck with a useless manager didn't help," Jack added reaching for another slice of pizza.

"When you're picked out of the crowd by one of the biggest rock stars on the planet, tour with a monster group like the Mac and get a song close to the Top Ten, you'd think you were all set," Stephan said as he aimed a half-eaten slice towards his mouth.

Jack explained that while Jiva got exposed to a large amount of the American public, getting dropped by the label turned off the money pipeline for promotion and touring. The sad part being that Alan could have pulled it off if he wasn't so worried about which party he was invited to next. If Alan had done his job, A&M records would have taken them over. When Polydor Records picked up the boys, the struggle for attention started all over again. Not only did they have to get the label to want to back them, the band also needed public support to generate the buzz that translates into label enthusiasm and more financial support as well as airtime on the local radio stations. LA is a huge market in itself and if a band can make it there, then the momentum would carry to the Midwest and East Coast as well.

"Before their tour, I gave them a new poem to work

into a song called 'Is It You' about searching for love in the crowded streets of a big city. It's less cynical than my earlier song 'One Out of Three'," Stephan said.

"It's a cool ballad, I like it. I guess after the Tania story, you found how to love again." Jack smiled at Stephan seeing he was able to make peace with the incident.

"Or at least believe in the possibility."

"I heard them jamming with it once so I wish you luck. Both with the song and the ladies. But as far as the band goes, it doesn't look like their spin of the wheel of fortune came up with a winner. But who knows." He shrugged his shoulders and took a swig of beer. "I hate to say it, but you may want to show your song to someone else, because I wouldn't count on them having a hit single with you or anyone else at this stage," Jack said.

"Understood. I only got enough royalty money from the first album to buy a six pack of beer."

Everyone resorted to a fallback plan and life returned to the normal pre-deal existence at Blem Gardens. Until a band hit the two to three gold record level, buying a condo at the beach was a remote possibility, much less a car with air conditioning and low miles. The only difference now was that Reedo, instead of working for a moving company, was the gardener for Stevie Nicks, the space queen singer from Fleetwood, who had a modern house out at the Marina Del Rey flatlands. He could wash her Jag and do a couple of lines here and there as a reminder of what was once the standard. The lead guitarist went back to carpentry building up-market recording studios, while Michael composed and sang jingles for radio commercials. Also, Jack got a new job as lab assistant to a commercial photographer, who was one of his desert rat buddies.

The fall from the heavens of rock and roll dreamland was hard, but the band's spirit wasn't broken. They were back doing gigs around town at smaller clubs again, yet somehow the fans' fervor had peaked. While the loyal diehards kept showing up, the buzz had moved on. Then one night, Reedo convinced Stevie to check out their recently reformed group that had a new guitar player and some hot tunes, in hopes that with her big solo success she might sponsor them or introduce the band to some of the music industry crowd she was adored by.

The gig was at a shabby neighborhood bar in Venice they had played a couple of times. It wasn't really a music place but the owner was accommodating enough to set up a small stage in a corner for them. It was a dead Monday night with a grey fog killing the enthusiasm of any potential audience members to venture out. There were more people in the band than in the audience and most of the public had only bought one drink in the first hour so the owner got offended and told the band to shut down as he wanted to go home.

Stevie showed up as promised around 9:30 with a couple of girlfriends, but found the place padlocked. It was the band's last gig.

20

HOME AWAY FROM HOME

James slipped his VW bus in the handicapped zone with only a tinge of guilt because it was the closest parking slot to the entry door. It was still dark and the valley hadn't woken up yet, with only a few cars on the streets indicating a gradual stirring human presence. A distant thumping like a faint heartbeat pulsated from the two-story building, where a row of lit windows beamed a welcome message to insomniacs and vampires. Inside, the programmers were coding away with the faint clacking of keyboards barely audible above the rock sounds blaring out of a pair of giant speakers hanging from the ceiling.

James walked the length of the room, thumping the walls of shoulder-high cubicles, where the core development team strung code together with an intense passion. Calling out a couple of names: "Hey, madman" or "What's up cuz?". He sat behind his desk in the corner office, flipping on his machine and while it booted up he shoved aside a pile of printouts to make room for a fresh stack. The company logo popped up on screen and soon James was joining the symphony of key clicks, with his own carefully picked-out tune called The Debugging Waltz.

James was fueled by ginseng-enhanced mu tea and unsalted rice cakes with the taste and consistency of the packing foam used to ship their computers. He had smeared the cakes with miso and tahini to manage his hunger and tapped through screen after screen of phosphorescent green characters. It was a day like any other, with random thoughts banished by the single-pointed goal the room hummed with. Only the feelings he had for Maria could break through the intense focus. James's mind flipped fitfully like a fish landed on a dock and took turns either mentally rationalizing it was okay she was gone because she smoked too much, drank espresso and ate sugar, while on the other hand missing her terribly, choking up with the fond memories of her smell and touch. The shock of her departure was settling in and he felt hollow and broken but he didn't know what to do. He thought he had been generous with his time and attention and didn't want to see that his definition of quality time didn't match Maria's. He shuffled from meeting to meeting with a heartache that he couldn't get rid of. There was a big hole in his life he kept feeling his way around and it amplified a deep sense of loneliness. He hadn't realized how close he had become with Maria and how much a part of his life she was, having in only a short while seeing the two of them as one entity. A part of him felt incomplete and broken. Work became his pain medicine. It only dulled the feeling as it was always there in the background, one thought away, waiting for the right moment to distract him with a tap on the shoulder.

Late nights, all-nighters and multiple days without sleep were necessary to meet the aggressive deadlines James pushed. And with this level of intensity he tried to forget Maria by filling in every waking moment with activity. His normal relentless work focus had been cranked up to a near manic level when the news broke that a couple of Yale dropouts who built the operating system for the IBM personal computers were hot on their tail, with a rival project to build the ultimate user interface.

Eden had pilfered the concept from the R&D labs of Xerox who didn't have commercial pretensions to sell the technology, as it wasn't related too much to their main product, photocopiers. The software used icons and boxes to contain work elements, and James had caught onto the potential in a split second. And while Eden was already showing a working prototype, the Yale guys who called themselves Microsoft were known to take no prisoners. Their CEO, Bill Gates would throw armies of programmers at a project and wanted to outdo Eden. Gates' user interface was clunkier and less elegant, which meant harder for the average user to work with, but their partner IBM was a standard setter, right or wrong.

James felt his vision of a people's computer was being hijacked, bastardized and sanitized. Market share came second to pride and winning the hearts and minds of his loyal customers and the general public, meant more than money, as it was about a vision. Microsoft wanted to step on him, the same way the Catholic Church had subjugated the early pagan tribes of nature worshipers and hijacking their images and holidays to bend them to their will. The possibility of being marginalized had gotten Grok back onboard. He was able to put past issues aside as the dreams

James promoted were also his own and he was back in his usual cubicle again.

James took a break to look for something different to smear on his Styrofoam-looking cake, hoping for an avocado. He lifted a shade and looked out the window of the break room for a second, pausing in a state of shock. With all the window shades in the long room having been lowered to keep out the day's eventual heat and contain the loud music blasting the neighbors, nobody had noticed that a convoy of tractors, semi-trucks and pickups were filling the parking lot and jamming the street.

A large flatbed truck pulled sideways across the parking lot, sporting a huge hand-painted sign that flapped with the activity, as if it were trying to shout its message:

EDEN IS DESTROYING THIS HEAVENLY VALLEY! EDEN GO TO HELL!

Just as he was reading the message out loud, the first apricot hit the building under where he stood, with a whopping noise. Teenaged kids standing in the back of a trailer had started hurling fistfuls of fruit at the offices. They looked like marauding Vikings intent on driving invaders out of their territory, without letting up until the last of the apricots had made their statement.

James and his team peeked out from under the curtains, fearful of what might happen next. Grok and another engineer joined James.

"Holy shit – this is insane!" Grok said.

"More than insane. Hey, Larry – call the police," James said to the other team member, a young guy with long hair wearing a Fillmore West T-shirt.

Larry said, "Looks like your girlfriend is getting her revenge."

"This isn't her style," he shot back. "I'm going down there to talk to them." James was like a protective mother and being outraged by the episode pushed whatever fear he had aside, wanting to protect his dream.

"Are you out of your mind – they'll tear you apart," Grok said as James stalked out of the office. Grok chased after him as fast as he could. "Hey, wait up!"

Grok and James walked out of the building, like two gunslingers facing down the bad guys at high noon, each not sure if they would be mobbed and beaten to a pulp. With James in the lead, they walked boldly towards the crowd as apricots continued to sail past them and smash against the building. James was irate and that overcame any fear of being hurt; he was defending his rights and more importantly his vision. The fruit stopped flying and the shouting quieted down. The farmers watched the two young men as they approached and stopped about thirty feet from the trucks.

James shouted to the crowd, "How many of you live in this valley?"

Someone from the mob scattered around the front of the trucks shouted back, "Fuck you!"

James wasn't fazed and tried to tone down the feelings of outrage while looking to set a diplomatic tone. "This valley is for all of us. There's enough room for everyone."

"Not if you tear down all the trees!" someone else screamed at them.

James responded, raising his voice to reach the entire

assembly, "I'm not after your farms. Ask the banks and developers to stop ripping you off. I make my money helping people, not stealing land." Grok looked around uneasily seeing that he and James were very exposed and no match for a large group of fit farm workers if a fight would break out.

The same person from the group of farmers responded and although it was loud, was an inch less aggressive than before, "Liar!"

"I'm getting all the tech companies together so we can work with you," James shouted back as he scanned the crowd making eye contact with a couple of young men.

In a car parked behind the farm wagons, the dead racer's father Roberto was watching. Sensing the crowd was starting to be swayed by the speech, he said something to one of his men leaning against the car. The man was holding a half-full bottle of beer and he suddenly turned and heaved it over the crowd in the direction of James and Grok. He then quickly picked up some fruit and started throwing it in the same direction, bellowing a war cry.

James was getting close to connecting with his audience. "We can start now—" but was cut off from his speech having to dodge the flying bottle and fruit. The crowd snapped out of their moment of quiet and started throwing fruit again while James and Grok ran back to their building, zigzagging to avoid being struck by flying projectiles. A handful of muscular young men led by the uncle's assistant gleefully started trashing a delivery van with the Eden logo on the side using sledgehammers and lengths of wood.

Maria had been in a funk for days after moving back to her parents' house. It was clear that in his current state of mind she couldn't live with James, but in her heart she knew that she couldn't live without him either. Her rational side would tell her it was all for the best and in time they could begin a new chapter. Mamacita consoled her, suggesting patience and was ready to play messenger if Maria decided to get in contact again.

Maria thought that perhaps if James had his fill of success and got it out of his system he would value her more and hopefully come to his senses sooner. She also knew that power and success was addictive as anything under the sun. The impending IPO had been hanging over James, a public vote of validation for his work and vision. One night Mamacita burst into her room clutching the evening *San Jose Mercury News*, with a big headline and pictures showing a riot at the Eden offices. The story mentioned how some irate farmers, including the Cappalettis, had organized a protest. Shocked by the event, she ran downstairs and found her father in front of the TV watching the news, having a beer before dinner.

"Papa, what is this?" Maria demanded, tossing the paper on a small table next to her father. "Has Roberto finally poisoned your mind?"

"Maria, this is not what it looks like."

"I know you don't approve of James but you didn't have to let Roberto smooth-talk you into supporting this ridiculous spectacle." She stood in front of him with her hands on her hips. "I feel sorry for you because you got deceived into making a fool of yourself."

"Now hold on a second—" Luigi eased himself upright from the depths of the Barcalounger, kicking the leg rest under the chair.

"Please hear me out. What about all the respect the farmers have for you? You're the one levelheaded person left in this valley. This riot makes you look reactionary and narrow minded." Maria quickly reached over and turned off the television then sat down firmly on the edge of the fireplace watching her father intently.

"Darling, try and see it from my eyes." Luigi sat forward in the armchair and put his beer on a low table. Concentrating on his daughter he spoke in a tired voice. "Not only am I losing my land and my heritage but I'm also losing my daughter. You represent the future and now I feel like a failure because my farms are disappearing and there's nobody else to pass this tradition on to."

"I know, Dad, how it must hurt you and it also makes me sad. But what happens to this valley has nothing to do with my love for James. He's not some land-grabbing maniac – he sincerely wants to help preserve the farms." Maria understood her father's pride and also regretted the potential passing of many generations of tradition.

"Look, I only want the best for you." There was a pause and then Luigi's words shifted to a more serious tone. "That's why for my sake you need to forget about this guy."

"Father, you're not being reasonable." Maria started to cry because for all his good intentions he was unable to separate James from the way the valley was evolving whether he liked it or not.

"I've never made more sense. There's been enough adventures lately and now it's time to get serious."

Maria spoke through her tears, her words breaking. "You're mixing up things here, don't you see? Each of these issues has their own causes and their own solutions. Trying to solve one with the other isn't going to work."

"I don't see it like that. Your boyfriend or whatever you call him is becoming one of the leaders of this new technology industry and that's his life. He's not an ecology type like he would want you to believe and his first love is his business, not an art student." Luigi reached for his beer and took a long swallow.

"That's not true." Her voice started to constrict and she wiped away some tears. "I don't know where you're getting these ideas but it's all wrong. I know him better than anyone and his talk about preserving the land is not a bunch of words just to make you happy. He really does have sensitivity for your situation. And yes, our relationship has been a bit rough lately but I still love him and I know he really loves me too."

"Then why did you move home if everything is so wonderful?" Luigi looked at his daughter with tired eyes.

"It's a respect thing. I know it's hard for you to understand but I support his vision and as you know the early days of building a business are the most demanding. James needs to have some time to focus and our time to be with each other was being compromised. So now we're taking a short breather and when that's over it will be better than ever." She said this proudly with all the certainty her young years could carry.

"I don't think the demands on your friend will ever be over. They'll only continue to grow and your so-called time-out won't end for a very long while." Luigi paused a second to look at her with a serious stare. He slowly got up out of the chair as if he was going to approach her. "Look, I just want you to be happy and I don't believe this guy is going to be the best for you in the long run. I'm your father, I know you so well and it's breaking my heart to see you put all your hopes and dreams into the hands of someone who doesn't care."

Maria got up quickly, stormed past her father and out of the room in a rage, running upstairs. She locked herself in her room, refusing to come down for dinner. With just the two of them at the dinner table, Maria's mother admonished her husband while she served the food. She could have been just off the boat from Rome dressed in a stylish bright print dress with her hair tied in a coil above her head.

"How can you be so cruel to Maria? Your flying off the handle like that isn't helping the situation."

"She won't listen if I don't stand my ground. That James fella has her brainwashed." Luigi started cutting his meat not looking her in the eyes.

"And DiFilippo didn't twist your thinking I suppose." Luigi looked up from his plate in reluctant acknowledgement. "You know that Maria is loyal to our family. She only wants what is best for you because it will be what is good for everyone. You can see she's in love, so please give her the chance to see where it can go. And if it isn't this James fellow it will be someone else but we need to support her, whatever she decides." Luigi's wife sat down and flipped open her napkin indicating her point was final.

Mamacita brought up a tray with some pasta, and she and Maria had a short chat. Later, when she was more composed, Maria got out the tarot cards as she did at key turning points of her life. Rather than do a full spread of the cards she decided to trust serendipity and shuffled the deck, randomly extracting one card from the middle. She turned it over – the card facing her was a skeleton on horseback, riding through a field of bodies – the card called Death.

The thirteenth card often spooked people, but Maria understood that it was symbolic of the death of one's lower self so the higher self could emerge. It indicated a time of change, and not literally a physical one, rather an indication of personal transformation.

She started to smile and picked up her phone to make a call. After about ten rings someone picked up on the other end.

"Hi Greg, it's Maria. I really need your help," she said in a fast-spoken mix of a command and cry for assistance.

"Hey, Miss Golden Goddess, slow down a sec. Is everything okay?" Greg said in a calming tone.

"Not at all. My father has totally flipped out. He and Roberto organized a riot at James's offices this morning." She gestured with her free hand as if Greg were in the room.

"Why'd he do that?" Greg said, surprised.

"He was convinced it would slow down construction in the valley."

"Then your old man has a new fulltime job. James is

not the only outfit growing like mad in that town." Greg's voice faded in and out momentarily as he moved around with the handset.

"And probably another motivation was to try and end my relationship with James once and for all because he doesn't want me to see him anymore." Maria's speaking had slowed down and took a more serious tone.

"I don't believe it. What can I do to help?" Greg's voice was clear and solid with a tone that said he was ready to do anything to support her.

"This is so cosmic. I just checked the tarot cards and I turned up the card of Death." Maria was toying with the card looking at it with a mischievous smile. "It gave me an idea – to end this life so I can start a new one."

"What?! Hey babe—" Greg was shocked and started to console her.

"I'm going to pretend I ran away to Europe so my parents will think I'm gone," she said with determination.

"God, you scared me. Maybe that's all you can do."

"It makes me a bit sad because I don't want to hurt them too much after Tobias's death."

"Yeah, everyone's still real emotional about that." At the sound of the racer's name Greg momentarily retreated into his guilt and there was an awkward silence for a second as Maria realized what she had said.

"I'll leave my car at the airport with a good-bye note and if it's okay with you, hide out at your place in Marin County." Maria reminded him that he had more than once offered her the use of his second home for yoga weekends or a painting retreat, so a personal getaway was a reasonable request.

"You're my most welcome guest. It's a perfect idea – nobody knows about my little hideaway." Greg's voice was lit up like he was a knight riding to a fair lady's assistance.

"The plan is to do it tomorrow morning so it looks like I'm going to school as usual. You can tell James where I am after I'm safe. I can never reach him because he's in meetings all the time."

"Cool. Let's hope your parents don't freak out too much," Greg said in a concerned tone sensitive to her family situation.

"Can we meet at nine in front of the departure area?"

"You can count on me!"

The next morning at the San Jose airport Maria parked her Fiat in the white loading zone in front of Departures. Greg pulled up behind her in his old Porsche and she quickly tossed her various bags and materials in his car and they drove off.

"With so many flights out of here it's going to take them weeks to figure out you didn't fly anywhere," Greg said smiling as they eased into the traffic on the freeway.

"By then I'll have made my point and my dad will see he can't control my life. It's so sweet of you to help." She reached over and squeezed his shoulder.

"Just doing my noble duty. And wait 'til you see this place. Stinson Beach is so cool. I first visited there with the Merry Pranksters for one of their parties."

"Sounds exotic," she said looking at him admiringly. "This is so nice of you – I'm really looking forward to having a private retreat."

"Yes, ma'am! You'll be right at home at my place. There's plenty of nature to inspire you," Greg said beaming, happy to see that his plans for the house as a hideout from civilization slowly started to become real.

Greg and Maria drove on Highway 101 along the bay, through San Francisco and crossed the Golden Gate Bridge. In Marin they drove down a stretch of Highway 1 by a long, wide beach before heading through the town of Stinson Beach and into the surrounding countryside. At the end of a winding dirt road they pulled up in front of a rustic cabin with an adjoining geodesic dome and distant view of the beach, and got out of the car.

"Home, sweet home! Other than a couple of crazy local chicks that are now lost and forgotten you are the first friend I've brought here," Greg said.

"I'm honored." She looked at the distant ocean. "This is incredible. I can't believe the view."

"C'mon, let me show you the layout and get you settled in."

They moved Maria's belongings into the cabin. She'd brought a couple of large drawing pads, a half a dozen blank canvases, an easel, paints and only a small suitcase for her clothes. Greg laughed at her packing saying she was the only woman he knew who didn't pack at least two major suitcases for a weekend. After unpacking some groceries, Greg made them some tea with peppermint from his backyard and explained how he had gotten the cabin cheaply from an old friend who was moving to Oregon. Using the drug money he'd previously earned in his days as Bernie's driver, he'd wanted to be able to live quietly and do his American sadhu in the country act. He even admitted he had come to the cabin a couple of times just to go cold turkey.

Greg took Maria out to the dome that he eventually intended to be a yoga room, part of a retreat for teaching yoga and the healing arts – Rancho Nirvana. Maria was touched by his dream and they sat on a beat-up old sofa in the dome enjoying the strange acoustics and ocean view.

"Greg, I love to hear you talk about your dreams like that. If you can dream something, it can become real. And I really see you one day having that beautiful center to help people. But dear one, you must really help yourself first." She looked at him over her mug of tea as she blew gently across the top to cool it.

"Yes, sweet angel, that's really true. And when I leave here today I'm heading to Big Sur to stay with a crazy Buddhist poet who's gonna straighten me out with mu tea and aduki beans, if you know what I mean. I'm going to do the big detox in a centered way to once and for all get me back to normal." Greg brought his hands together in a namaste prayer position and bowed his head slightly to show the holiness of his intent.

"Oh, Greg I really wish you can finally do it. I know it's such a hard thing to break away from." Maria reached over and touched him on the arm briefly.

"It's is the proverbial monkey on the back to be sure. And 'cause cold turkey is so godawful bad, once you're clean and the shakes and shits are over and hallucinations all gone you feel you should be rewarded for all the hell you intentionally suffered through. One little hit sure looks like the sweetest reward for working through all the pain."

"I know it's hard, but please promise me that this time you'll really try because you want to control it and not be controlled by it. It's your choice to live and you don't need drugs to appreciate life."

"Wiser words were never spoken, sweet lady of the Tarot and princess of the paints. I think I've given Gloria too much of an excuse to ignore me when I'm strung out. Heard she might be seeing another fella. That little darlin' schoolteacher cousin of yours sure ain't someone I want to lose touch with, if you know what I mean."

Maria nodded sagely with a big grin. "And do me a favor – wait a little while before you tell James where I am. I want to have some time for myself and I think he needs to find his heart and rediscover that fire to make our crazy world work."

"You got it, baby."

Greg hustled about preparing the cabin for Maria and put on the Lynyrd Skynyrd album *Street Survivors* and when it came to a live version of the song 'Free Bird' Greg sang along:

If I leave here tomorrow
Would you still remember me?
For I must be traveling on, now
'Cause there's too many places I've got to see
But if I stayed here with you, girl
Things just couldn't be the same
'Cause I'm as free as a bird now
And this bird you cannot change

And this bird you cannot change

Maria was listening from the front lawn and had a sudden premonition that chilled her but she didn't know what it meant. The image of the original album cover stuck in her mind – a picture of the band engulfed in flames. A few months before the record was released a couple of the band members had died when their tour plane crashed and the album cover had to be changed from the one with the fire to one with a plain black background. She assumed the image was echoing James's recurring nightmare from India he had shared with her but at the same time she was also praying it wasn't going to be the good-bye message James would eventually play for her as a result of her actions.

Soon after Maria's disappearance word got back to James via the valley grapevine and the news stopped him in his tracks. His first reaction was to worry if she was safe, not knowing the exact circumstances of her leaving. He had no one he could call because her parents wouldn't talk to him, much less share anything with him, and as Gloria wasn't reachable when he tried phoning her, he was left to his own anxieties. At the same time, he was again regretting his actions that had driven her away and wished he could turn back the clock to reset his behavior. The sting of the good-bye slap was burning his cheek again.

21

BAD, BAD MELVIN BROWN

Anthropologists have been able to determine that Neanderthal humanoids coexisted for a time with Cro-Magnon man, the ancient relatives of today's humans. But if these same scientists wanted proof that the two species intermingled and survived they would have to look no further than Melvin. He had a head that bore a striking resemblance to King Kong, with a square jaw, close-cropped hair and slanted forehead above deep-set eyes. The face said 'I'm primitive', most likely crude even, but also calculating (if using fingers to help count were allowed) and definitely menacing.

The jungle he inhabited stretched a couple of streets north of Interstate 10, west to around Culver City, east to within a mile of downtown and south as far as Inglewood. The center of action was around Western and 153rd Street, the middle of South Central. Not to be confused with a ghetto, there were respectable family houses struggling to remain in lower middleclass status on the streets crossing Western. Working mom-and-pops and kids going to school with *Sesame Street* lunchboxes mainly occupied the modest homes.

After dark the area transformed itself into locked, shuttered fortresses where only the creatures of the night prowled. A lot of dusters hung out on the street corners along Western. These were the bored black youths, smoking angel dust. They were frying an already uneducated brain, so that their more Neanderthal traits surfaced: smash and grab, smack the bitch, smoke that shit. Dust was a variety of elephant tranquilizer, sprinkled on mint leaves and smoked in tiny joints the size of a toothpick. The dose was incredibly potent, with immediate intense hallucinations and feelings of rapture. In some cases it triggered extreme violent reactions that were hard for police to restrain as the drug lowered the mental limitations of the user, giving the illusion of superhuman strength. The behavior of the dusters was unpredictable and even the most minute circumstance could trigger a brutal response. Something trivial could set them off, like a lone white kid cruising their territory at one in the morning.

Melvin's house was in the middle of a block of modest homes with small front yards boxed in by low chain-link fences and screen doors with the glow of a TV shining through. By associating with white people like Stephan, Melvin scored points in the eyes of his neighbors. Melvin would call Stephan to make a delivery in the early afternoon during the week when nobody was around except the other unemployed parents or else early morning like 1 a.m. or so when the dusters were dusted and had mostly crawled back under their rocks.

'Come on, little birdie' was the friendly invite, as it was all upbeat with Melvin, as he had respect for Miami Will and his buddies for some unknown reason. Perhaps it was something to do with their being Vietnam vets, not afraid to use firepower when the occasion warranted. The deals always went down quick and the product and price were always consistent. Five hundred a pound, five pounds at a time, exchanged for a stack of well worn, grubby twenties. Sometimes Melvin would offer designer jeans in trade that had fallen off the back of a truck or some such shit. Stephan wasn't sure if he should be more afraid of the cops when he was carrying or the street punks and gangbangers. Being the only white guy for five square miles made him stand out like a chicken in a fox's den to both sets of eyes.

Melvin was continually frustrated at being unable to buy cocaine and never failed to ask, in case he could find an opening. Eventually he started to try and shortchange Stephan on the count, with the added distractions of beautiful black girls in short shorts cavorting around, while R & B music played and the Jack Daniels got poured. Usually it was a friend of Mel's wife who would just happen to be around, with smiles and cleavage that said 'take me home – you won't be sorry' and other than a little conversation, Stephan was able to focus on the business at hand.

Stephan hadn't really caught on to Melvin's tactics, but still managed to come away regardless with the correct amount of money even though it meant recounting it several times. He had been warned that not even the blacks trusted the blacks, so what chance did he have. And then things started to go slowly wrong. Sometimes not all the money was there and Stephan would end up with a late-night round-trip, carrying shit both directions, which was less than ideal. Driving into the middle of the black ghetto in the wee hours of the morning with a sports sack of drugs meant that either the police or local gangs would have fun if they checked him. Having to repeat the journey twice with the contraband was more than nerve-wracking.

When the call came one Saturday afternoon, the drop was at a new location, some house deeper into South Central off of Western that Stephan had never been to before. Stephan blasted down the near empty Santa Monica Freeway, driving east from the beach and exited at Western, heading south. The cross streets were getting higher and higher in number and at every intersection, groups of blacks hanging out would study him like some foreign creature. Not only were the idle youths in baggy sports clothes or girls in miniskirts staring, but the older people as well, who were carrying bags of groceries. Stopped at a signal, he was afraid for a second of getting robbed, but the light would always mercifully change before any of the locals could rally up and move in on him.

Turning down the designated street of run-down two-story houses, he spotted the house number part way down the block and parked in front. Stephan couldn't believe that this beat-up house needed a ten-foot high chain-link fence to keep out the invisible crowd off the street. As soon as Stephan was out of his car, Melvin appeared, waving from the back of a dirt drive that went down the left side of the house, outside the fence. Stephan hefted his sport sack and trudged along, while Melvin motioned for him to hurry. Any rival gang driving by would have guessed the action and tried to muscle in with their friends, Mr. Smith and

Mr. Wesson or Mr. Remington and their European cousins Herr Glock and Herr Ruger.

The deal went down on the kitchen table of the whorehouse. Stephan had entered the small room through a short hallway from the backdoor. No sooner than he was seated, sweet soul sisters teased him and brought over ice cold beers sweating with condensation. Melvin was the master of ceremonies, playfully swatting the girls away if they got too close to the stacks of twenties he was spreading on the table. Floral perfume wafted in the air as the girls sashayed around.

A minute later Melvin was offering Stephan his choice of ladies. "Ain't she fine? Sweet Samantha wanna play with your tool, man," breaking into a raucous laughing fit, slapping him on the back.

On cue, Samantha would drape her arm over Stephan's shoulders, a large, firm breast tickling his ear, while a flat belly grazed his bare arm, making his hairs stand on end. Her Moulin Rouge cousin, also in denim hot pants, wore an electric blue, striped top that left no part of the anatomy to the imagination. She would gyrate to the blaring R & B music and prop a leg on a chair, suggestively slipping her fingers into the top of her cut-off jeans that showed the nice crease of her ass. She then withdrew them, to slide them into her mouth like they were covered with Colonel Sanders' 'finger lickin' good' Kentucky Fried Chicken seasoning. The lazy motion would be accompanied by a sultry stare that would break into a big, toothy smile before she moved off and bounced around to the music some more.

It took four tries at recounting the money to get the

count right, and the party had grown. Each time Melvin would push the piles of worn twenties in front of him, Stephan would double-check the amount but it was never the full sum. Melvin would protest and insist the money was all there and the girls would look on, like Stephan was the guilty party.

Beers were flowing, each one sliding down easier than the previous, the music booming and the sweet ladies danced around and strutted their long legs. They seductively swayed their high, fine asses or bent over in their spandex tube tops with ample breasts begging to pop out, nipples pointing through, just waiting for a tweak. He was the man, the one, could have even had a couple of the fine young girls at the same time to play with. Melvin kept encouraging him, and the ladies went wild seeing so much cash in one place, especially in the hands of a john who could be gotten drunk and rolled for most of it inside of an hour.

In the end, Melvin was seven hundred short and begged Stephan to leave all the grass so his partners and regular customers wouldn't get too upset. Besides, Melvin rationalized, "You don't want to drive home with this load."

The primitive look said: 'you won't even make it to your car and if you do, you won't get too far'. A pump action shotgun leaning against the refrigerator also indicated the area might not have been as friendly as desired, even in broad daylight. Stephan was confused from smoking too much Hawaiian on the drive over and being a few beers over his limit. He slowly realized he was outnumbered and would even be lucky to get out of the blasted house with any money or product at all. He gave in reluctantly to a round of cheers from the girls. Stephan was unaware he was getting sloppy with his business affairs from increased coke use from club sojourns with The Count, and ever more powerful joints that dulled his awareness.

Melvin pulled the same stunt a second time a couple of weeks later. With his smooth-talking ghetto jive and Stephan's 1 a.m. paranoia, he got into Stephan for another eight hundred. Now Stephan was out fifteen hundred, with no hope in sight of recouping the money. The next week's delivery was a chance for payback.

Turning the tables on Melvin, Stephan asked for half the money up front, justifying the excuse by blaming it on his supplier who wasn't happy. Miami Will, had he been informed, would have simply made a phone call and the outstanding cash would have appeared the next day, but this hadn't occurred to Stephan. He met Melvin in the parking lot of an In-N-Out Burger shop off La Cienega, under the shadow of Interstate 10. Stephan took the twelve fifty in cash and never went back at the appointed time. When Stephan checked his answer machine, Melvin had left five messages. The first was a curious and confused query and they got gradually more desperate, so by the third or fourth call it was a pleading, whining, begging Melvin, claiming his customers would be all over him. Stephan knew Melvin didn't know where he lived, but he wasn't too comfortable knowing that half of South Central would be looking to nail his ass.

Stephan was getting Out There, where normalcy was a thing of the past. He was dating a new lady, a curvaceous blond French girl named Yvette he met at one of Harry's parties who was teaching modern dance in a studio at the beach. Stephan thought that a down-to-earth lady with old world values might be the counterbalance to his life that was gradually slipping into a permanent haze, rationalized by believing that he was becoming another roaming angel bohemian like Greasy, spreading cool wherever he went. The French lady initially thought Stephan was selling vitamins when he made his drops and when she found out the truth it didn't matter, as he was gentle, articulate and caring. Her naiveté was refreshing, but sometimes her emotions got out of hand in loud explosions of irrational outbursts only a French artist could express with authenticity without looking like they were an escapee from a lunatic asylum. But life was stressful enough so it became clear after a few dates a high-strung French import wasn't compatible to his getting along with what he had to deal with. After a serious discussion with her about eternal friendship, brother and sister closeness and how they would always remain friends, Yvette soon headed north to teach at a community college.

One minor benefit from the adventure was that Lila had suddenly gotten more interested in Stephan when she saw him sliding towards a relationship in his early dating with Yvette. Up until then, there hadn't been any serious ladies in his life and with a sixth sense that only women possess, Lila could see the makings for a possible permanent liaison. She went with him for a coffee after yoga class one night in a small student bar in Westwood while Yvette was staying with him. They found an empty booth and after a laugh about Bilkem's latest girlfriend and an update on her screen pursuits, she turned philosophical.

"I think that what we believe to be real is our own creation. It starts all the way down in our emotions. The world is like a neutral screen and we project onto it our own experience. When I'm happy, the whole world is happy and when I'm down, the world looks pretty bleak." Lila was playing the role of a philosopher knowing this type discussion would interest Stephan.

"I agree. We are the ones that make the good and bad," Stephan said as he picked up his iced tea and took a drink.

"Like in the movies. The screen is blank until the projector displays whatever roll of film is loaded in it. So Mr. Party Guy, are you still managing to find the truth in your life movie, or is the adrenaline rush from dodging cops and robbers now the real buzz?" Lila said as she reached for her herbal tea.

"Thanks for asking. Maybe the excitement is attractive, and my all too rational mind can justify the adventures as material for my book, but even so the writing is lagging."

"You can't forget your focus, not even for a second 'cause that's all it takes to spin out of control," Lila said in a motherly tone.

"You must be my guardian angel, besides being the sweetest goddess this side of nirvana." Stephan blew her a kiss across the table. She smiled broadly at the compliment. "Are you okay? The work scene not getting you down?"

"No more than usual. But you know what? After all the hyper yoga chakra crunching workout, my lower back is hurting. You think there's any chance of getting one of your world-famous back rubs?" Lila asked innocently.

Stephan initially hesitated, but that lasted about a tenth of a second before he agreed, having spun through in that split second a thousand thoughts about blocked chakras, French lovers, commitment, love for this lady and his little brain saying 'go for it'. Lila suggested they go back to his place and as Yvette was teaching a class out at the beach, there was some privacy. No sooner had they gotten to his bungalow, Lila led the way into the bedroom and lay down on his thick oriental rug. She wiggled out of her T-shirt, unzipped her jeans, pulling them down halfway over her ass, and lay on her belly waiting expectantly. Stephan practiced his utmost self-control and some almost audible breaths to keep the massage on a purely healing level, although the invitation to go further had never before been so available. He was sorely tempted to make a move, but a sense of duty or honor, respecting Yvette, kept his intent pure. There was lust in his heart nonetheless. To distract his focus from his wandering intentions Stephan talked about helping Maceo pitch his script and reminded her again of the story and how she would make a perfect Indian princess that received a sensually delivered positive Native American inspired 'ummm' in response.

Lila was grateful for the massage and kissed him quickly on the mouth before she left. Half an hour later, Yvette returned, to find the steamy funk from Lila's body still hanging in the air. While the two ladies knew each other, Yvette was wondering if Stephan was having an affair. Being French, it didn't rate high on reasons to start a fight, and Stephan was insistent nothing had transpired so she was content. Somehow Lila was attempting to mark her territory, even though she lacked the courage to fully claim it in an honest show of emotion.

Just to make life more interesting, another customer, the Lebanese Mafia was also pushing now. Their front man, Duane, worked for PacBell at their Redondo Beach switching center and with a couple of internal directory queries on information the public couldn't access, Duane located Stephan's bungalow and dropped by one night to say 'hi'. Stephan immediately knew that whatever product he had wouldn't be secure anymore. Terms and conditions would be negotiated in Duane's favor and no privacy or security would remain.

The scary thing was these Lebanese guys were hard-core cases. On one visit to Duane's shabby Redondo Beach apartment, the squat Lebanese garage owner with the perpetual three-day stubble told a story he thought was funny as hell. Maybe it was a warning not to mess with them or perhaps it was really only their idea of a good time.

"There's this guy that crossed us and to let him know we weren't happy, we sent him to the hospital. And just to remind him we don't forget our friends, we were waiting in the parking lot for the guy when he got released, and broke his arm again." The garage owner was laughing hysterically and demonstrated how it was done by taking Stephan's arm and holding it over his knee, pretending to break it, like snapping a small piece of wood in half. Big laughs, funny shit, eh? Stephan had laughed along like it was the funniest joke he had ever heard, realizing these guys were psychotic. Now they knew where he lived, they would be visiting whenever they pleased, whether he was there or not.

The weirdness continued when the Righteous Reverend, a black Evangelical hell raiser, complete with Cadillac stretch limo, had disappeared after getting into him for a couple of hundred worth of assorted goodies. Visits to the cousin who had introduced them, a session player he met through the band, only provided a 'moved, no forwarding address' note on the mailbox and a pool of dry blood in the hallway. Stephan didn't feel up to visiting every Bible thumping congregation in South Central to track him down, so it was another write-off.

It was about this moment in time Miami Will came for a visit, because due to some funny bookkeeping it looked like Stephan had pocketed a few grand, even though it was just a case of general incompetence. Numbers were never Stephan's strength and while he thought he was keeping accurate records, Will had been counting kilos and Stephan had been counting dollars and a discrepancy gradually developed after a couple of months. They hadn't caught up to the recent deals otherwise Melvin's shortchanging would have been obvious. Stephan's pride made him sure he could make it up and didn't want to anger Will.

Stephan called Will where he was staying at Brandi's new apartment by the beach and sorted out the problem. The call was awkward at first as Will wasn't sure if Stephan really was ripping him off or not. They talked as usual using cryptic code words as Will was paranoid about using the public phone system. Kilos became yards of lumber and blond wood was Colombian gold. They sorted out the differences when Stephan's lack of bookkeeping skills became obvious and agreed on a number. At this point something nasty was bound to happen, the karmic forces were swirling too thick not to cause some effect.

The life raft bouncing on the ocean of madness was the ever-progressing script, as the Ronarama story (as the novel was now called) was now collecting dust. The motivating aspects that helped Stephan keep up his meditation and inner focus were gone, replaced by other supporting factors of a more transitory nature. Since Lila had hooked them up with Bob, Stephan and Mac had been working every free moment to bend the screenplay to Bob's taste. Bob kept asking for changes to make it more showable, because he rationalized that before he could put it in front of someone who could green-light it, the script should be in the best possible shape as there was only one chance to make a big first impression.

Bob constantly dropped names and bragged about whom he had lunch with at Ma Maison, to keep the team fired up. He repeatedly assured the two partners he could land fifty grand in development money to get the story really in shape as soon as he had a decent script. Mac and Stephan worked long into the night for weeks and the script bounced back and forth like a tennis ball at the US Open.

The three of them had frequent meetings at a coffee shop down the street from Blem Gardens on Santa Monica Boulevard that eventually made Stephan suspicious, as

Bob had his own office at the studio. Bob always appeared dressed in black and to match his heavy gold chain around his neck he wore a massive bracelet that he rattled on the table. He always smelled like he had splashed on a gallon of Paco Rabanne cologne. When he wasn't being chauffeured, he drove his custom Porsche with racing stripes that looked out of place in the shabby diner's parking lot. But he was enthusiastic and kept the lads pumped up. Bob took the latest draft along on a Friday to read over the weekend and said he would get back to them. A week later there was no word from him and they got worried. No calls were returned and after a second week had passed a UPS package arrived with the story enclosed and no cover letter. The sender on the label was Bob's production office. Mac and Stephan were shocked and even Lila couldn't get on Bob's calendar anywhere to obtain some feedback.

A few days later Stephan was at a party in Beverly Hills with one of his clients, a lady accountant, and met her hairdresser, a stylish guy in his fifties who claimed to be the basis for the character Warren Beatty played in the film *Shampoo*. Every hairdresser in the Hills made this claim.

They got into some macho posturing and the hairdresser claimed his grass was better than Stephan's private stash from Humboldt County and dared him to guess the source. Next, they bragged about their movie business contacts and whose hair he had done versus Stephan's rock star stories. When the subject got around to films, Stephan started in on his screenplay and the hairdresser started laughing.

"You'll never believe this. I was doing a guy's hair a couple of days ago and he told me about your film."

"What?" Stephan said as he exploded a lungful of smoke.

"Yeah, in fact he said he was able to get the studio to agree to an exclusive first look option for one week and they agreed. Got a hundred grand for the privilege, if you can believe the guy." The hairdresser took a slow, cool draw on his drink.

"I don't believe it."

"The guy's name was Sampson, like in the Bible; black outfits, gold hardware," the hairdresser said.

"That's him all right, but what's this bullshit?" Stephan related his story and the hairdresser looked at him like he was a complete fool.

"You had no agent or contract?"

"No, we were acting on good faith," Stephan said.

"Good luck, there's not much you can do legally," the man said shaking his head sadly.

After none of his calls to Bob were returned and all he could get was increasingly rude brush-offs from the secretary, Stephan camped out in front of the studio waiting for the guy. The security guard was suspicious and wrote down his license number. When Bob finally appeared one hour later in the Porsche with the top down, Stephan followed him and at the first stoplight pulled up next to him and started a shouting match. When Stephan threatened to contact the studio, the producer laughed.

"I have my own arrangements and what's between you and me is of no concern to the studio, so forget about it," Bob shouted.

"What if I tell them about all the grass I sold you?"

"You want me to admit I'm a drug user and you're a dealer? Give me any shit and I'll drop the dime. The police would be happy to get scum like you off the streets."

The cars behind had started honking as the light had changed, so the producer gunned the Porsche. Bob raised his right hand, giving Stephan the finger, as he sat in his beat-up Honda fumbling with the stick shift with his eyes stinging from the stink of Bob's burning rubber.

22

THE WRONG PLACE AT THE RIGHT TIME

Venice by night was a no man's land. Black gangbangers like the Crips and Bloods had their turf battles with Hispanic Mafia units like the Bluesmen and the Undertakers, amidst an assortment of junkies, winos, dusters and mental cases, all scurrying around like fearless cockroaches in a dark Miami kitchen. Even a black-and-white cruiser with a couple of LAPD's finest had a minimal effect on the scene. Both sides generally ignored each other in an uneasy truce, until the next drive-by shooting.

Stephan was sitting in a broken-down house from the fifties that had probably been pretty decent in its prime, when it was a comfortable middle-class home. It was keeping some other past their sell-by date haciendas company, along a forgotten residential section of Rose Avenue, about four blocks in from the beach.

Stephan had decided to break his golden rule – don't mess with coke. The random violence and high risks had kept him away from this world until now. Even when The Count had asked Stephan to fly to Chicago with him to bring a few ounces to the Eagles for one of their infamous Third Encore parties while touring to promote

Hotel California, he turned him down. And now Stephan had recently started to consume it when offered, and even bought the occasional gram, but considered it an extravagance. He had thought using coke would give him the energy to complete his story and increase his creative output, but the drugs nature only made him create freakier scenes where the demons were more evil and bloodthirsty than even the original Ramayana expressed.

He felt good naturally, so grinding teeth, sweaty palms and a nervous mind didn't carry much appeal when compared to the laid-back high from some bright green Maui Wowee or stinky Humboldt skunk. The grass better suited his modern contemplative style, now that mindful breathing and yoga postures were too time-consuming.

Miami Will's calculations led him to figure out Stephan owed him for quite a few pounds. And while Will had offered to extend the arrangement with Stephan after the previous driver had decided to add some extra weeks to his round-the-world trip, it was important to keep the balance up to date. Stephan had given Bob Sampson some cut-rate prices and had also traded a couple of quarters for coke, to keep Bob on the job of pushing the screenplay. With what Melvin had shorted him and Bob's skipping out it left Stephan holding the bag (or empty baggie as it were). The grass business wasn't expanding and without Melvin as a big regular customer was even shrinking, so there weren't too many alternatives left to raise some quick cash.

Desperate situations require desperate actions, so Stephan took the plunge. Having gone far enough down the new path that he had eventually gotten lost on, turning back wasn't a consideration to his cloudy thinking. Since his last visit with Greg, a sense of resignation had set in that made wanting to walk the high road once again feel like self-righteous posturing. Whenever he thought of Greg, he felt sad and helpless, with a touch of complicity. The doubt machine was back in gear again, and his fears of being unable to complete his Ronorama project or find a receptive audience were compounded by wondering if he couldn't help a friend in need, how could he help anyone else, much less himself. Best to ride it out and let the cosmos bring him to where he should be. All is change, so if he waited long enough, all this would pass. He felt he had hit the bottom, so the only place left to go was to head back up. The first step would be to relieve some of his debts.

One big coke deal would score enough cash to get Will off his back. If it went well, he would scale another two or maximum three increasingly larger deals, to get enough cash to leave dealing altogether. He would be able to set up his own small publishing business and support his writing efforts and he could start a new life. Like all dealers looking for freedom from their self-imposed secret world, he was sure that this would be it, one last big deal, the big deal in the sky to end it all.

His grass contacts had been pestering him constantly for blow and so he started out with the Lebanese in Redondo. He had brought them a tasty eighth of an ounce to whet their appetite that they gladly bought. It was a sample of what a quarter pound would be like. With Stephan as the middle man, he could make on the high end, fifteen to twenty thousand and after a couple of deals of escalating size would be done with it – out of there, finished, adios amigos. He remembered how easy Greasy had made it look: be cool and talk the talk, massage it with a little jive and keep all parties happy so they would have some trust and do repeat biz.

The Count was away on an extended vacation for a few weeks with a South African lady, so Stephan worked with two guys in Venice, who sold him the sample. He knew them from hanging out at the beach, as they were also friends of The Count. Being Latinos with a direct contact to the source south of the border, they could get any amount of cocaine he wanted. They talked about boats stopping off Catalina after a cruise to Mexico and offloading cargos of duffle sacks to waiting pleasure craft. The smaller boats then headed back home to Marina Del Rey, with a hardcore crew below decks and M14s with the safety off, set to automatic, not single shot.

Ray and José were cousins, with family in the Puerto Rican community in New York City. Ray was the more tasteful dresser and preferred sta-pressed slacks and a polyester shirt with modern patterns and pointed collars, while José was the sporty type with a Lakers sweatshirt and jeans. They had partied on several occasions when Stephan would skate over after cruising the Venice boardwalk. Their house had a family feel, as it was home to a revolving cast of relatives staying in their guest room.

On this particular night, Stephan was going to talk about setting up a deal with the Lebs for a quarter pound, as a trial run for a full pound. Stephan and the cousins were getting mellow behind some good grass and uncut flaky toot, with a good discussion going on about the ups and downs of their business. Stephan had taken a break from the living room to chat with their most recent guest, a teenager who was taking some classes at the local junior college. The kid was the son of a friend back east, that made him part of the family and a welcome guest. Stephan had told him about the book he was writing and shared some words from his meeting with the silent baba before rejoining the living room party. The student was intrigued by the stories and they agreed to talk more about yoga one afternoon later in the week.

There was a knock at the door and José said it's just a couple more beach bums like you, nodding to Stephan, who looked anxious with a cocaine nervousness amplified by the grass. José opened the door and two black men in their early twenties sauntered in. One was dressed in a running suit with a sports bag casually slung over his shoulder, while the other wore baggie overalls and a tank-top T-shirt showing off bodybuilder arms with tattoos all over, the most prominent being the Chicago Bulls logo on a buffed-out bicep.

"Yo, bro. What's up?" Ray said.

"Not much," the sporty one in Fila gear answered.

José came round the sofa after securing the door and invited them to sit down. He took his place at the low living room table in front of the mirror and started to chop up some small rocks.

"Wanna do a line?" José asked glancing up at the two visitors.

Before an answer came, the sportsman reached into his

bag and pulled out a sawed-off shotgun.

"Yeah, we want some coke, but not that piddly ass shit. Give us your main stash, asshole."

Stephan looked at the man's face and saw his eyes were vacant of any signs of life, almost obliterated by bloodshot veins crisscrossing them like intricate spider webs. The muscleman projected a nervous tension like a vicious dog, rabies-crazed and unpredictable. If Stephan's heart had been pounding earlier, it was hammering loudly now, so that his temples were throbbing. The adrenaline kicked in, but with no flight possible, fright took over.

The two cousins said to take it easy and while sporty guy held the gun on José and Stephan, the partner retrieved a silver automatic pistol out of the sports sack and went with Ray through all the rooms to see the layout. Finally, they disappeared into one of the bedrooms and came out a minute later with a baggie that Stephan reckoned must have been a couple of ounces of coke, as it was about four fingers thick. It was double bagged, the bulk evident. They had left the student sleeping.

"That's all we've got, swear to god," Ray said.

The Fila man grunted and motioned with the shotgun for Ray to join José on the sofa. While the Bulls man stood by, Mr. Fila said, "I don't want any shit so I'm going to leave you with a warning." He went back to the bedroom where the student was sleeping and then they all heard a muffled boom, startling all of them, except the Bulls fan.

Fila came back and said, "Don't even think of coming after us," and as quickly as they had arrived, they were gone into the night, with the front door left open and the screen door banging hollowly against its cheap metal frame.

The two cousins and Stephan rushed back to the bedroom. Stephan managed to see over the cousins' shoulders, where they crowded around the bed. The student lay face up under the covers with a gentle expression and a big, dark red spot about six inches wide across the middle of his belly. The smell of the gunpowder had faded and there was another more clinical smell that Stephan didn't register at first. It caught in his throat like the taste of something metallic. Then it dawned on him it was the smell of blood, like when he stood in front of the butcher counter in the market.

Stephan went into shock and all he could say was, "Oh my god, oh my god," with the emphasis shifting from one word to the next with each repetition as tears streamed down his face. The scene of senseless violence he was witness to but unable to do anything about momentarily triggered a flashback from India of the innocent girl who had been burned alive while he stood by helplessly.

José and Ray cursed and cried and insisted Stephan should leave immediately, because they had to clean up the paraphernalia and call the police. Stephan stumbled into the bathroom and heaved over the toilet with nothing coming up except bile that burned his throat. Stephan was still in shock when he found his way back to the living room. José grabbed him, telling him again to leave right away, as the police were coming and not to take his car otherwise the neighbors would think he was part of the set-up – come and get it tomorrow, José suggested.

Stephan managed to find his way out the door on his shaky legs, and then getting his bearings straight, walked as best he could down the sidewalk away from the beach wiping away tears and putting on a brave face. The uneven cement slabs were strewn with trash and some worn-out palm trees on either side hung on to their dusty existence. He spotted a lit-up Pac-Tel logo on top of a payphone at the next corner by a Mexican restaurant in the direction of Lincoln Boulevard and shuffled along to make a call.

23

THE LAND THAT TIME FORGOT

James was leaning against a large boulder on the mountain ridge overlooking the Santa Clara Valley. It was the usual retreat when contemplating serious matters or else spacing out and letting the universe flow. The native Indians had used it for similar purposes so the energy was retained for subsequent generations. James was smoking a fat joint while gazing intently at a photo of Maria. He ignored the cold fog blowing by that made everything damp and gloomy. A false sense of warmth was created by a bottle of Jack Daniels and a baggie full of assorted drugs. With only a denim jacket for cover he needed to dip into the liquor and drugs to keep from freezing. James started speaking out loud as if he was having a conversation with Maria, his words slightly slurred from lack of sleep and assorted substances swirling on his brain.

"Baby, I miss you. Why is it I'm always saying I'm sorry? But you know I love you." He put the joint down and took a swig of Jack. "I don't believe you went far away. Our love is too perfect."

He had been in a state of shock and emotionally punched in the stomach since hearing two days before that Maria had run away from home. When a mutual friend from the local paper had told him Maria's car had been found at the airport with a good-bye note he had immediately taken the blame for her leaving. The note had mentioned her love for him and hoped that one day they could be together. James had left the office immediately when he heard the news, gathering up a smorgasbord of drugs from the various engineers. He wanted to blot out his sorrow and regret, not wanting to break down in front of his staff and at the same time was wondering where she could have gone. The note had mentioned Italy but somewhere inside his intuition told him otherwise. His emotions were too tangled-up between his love for Maria and the waves of guilt that broke over him relentlessly to have any clarity. The first wave was the handling of his relationship and seeing what a self-centered fool he had been when presented with the perfect partner. This triggered the resulting wave of guilt over how he had been ignoring his friend Greg when he needed help and then the last wave was the race. They would all repeat in random order, washing over his shattered feelings the drugs and alcohol exaggerated. The business issues became irrelevant and he felt he had nothing to prove anymore, thinking he was a world-class hypocrite to preach harmony and enhanced human potential. He had been in this state for two days, the first night passing out in his bus in a redwood forest near the coast. Later he found his way to the mountaintop, as his inner compass brought him to a place where maybe his situation could be clarified or else turn seriously bad.

James squeezed his eyes tightly shut as if the concentrated

pressure would blow away the confusing thoughts. He kept his eyes closed and took a deep breath to try and center as best as his condition would allow. His rational mind had a second to step up as the emotions regrouped for creating a bigger set of more guilty waves. In slow motion James looked logically at all the possible alternatives to Italy. His shattered brain had to back up a couple of times to refocus on the option he was thinking about. The cousin in Santa Cruz was one possibility but he had ruled that one out when he had passed by the house early in his two-day binge and found an equally mystified Gloria. He stepped through a mental list of school friends but was sure Marie wouldn't hide in plain sight. Maybe the family had a vacation house he didn't know about and she had sneaked off to hide out there. As he struggled to think up more items to add to the mental checklist the last idea hadn't entirely faded from his consciousness and echoed in another corner of his brain. The getaway home thought linked via a wobbly neural pathway to a similar distant memory of hearing Greg had acquired a hideaway in his saner days as a basis for a yoga retreat. The slumbering brain cells suddenly lit up in a cluster of flashes and clanging bells like hitting the jackpot on a Las Vegas slot machine.

James heard a car approaching from the north on the two-lane Skyline Boulevard at the base of the ridge. He raised his groggy head and peered through the fog with faint interest. It was a new Porsche 911 that raced by and quickly disappearing down the road, accelerating on the straightaway. It was a sign from the depths of the synchronistic universe that his hunch was right.

"Greg! I knew it – you're hiding out with that bastard. Son of a bitch!"

James tossed the whiskey bottle away and it made a painful clinking sound against the rocks. He pushed himself up; stiff from the cold and awkward position he had been sitting in. He stumbled down the rough hillside towards his bus parked along the road below. A couple of minutes later James was standing in a phone booth at the edge of a parking area for a scenic viewpoint on the corner of Highway 9 with a blue box hooked up to the handset.

Uncertainty had become the only certainty for Stephan. He was more paranoid than usual as the killers of the Puerto Ricans' houseguest were still at large. Fear of going to jail for dealing had been replaced with the waking nightmare of another possible visit by some gangbanger homeboys who were friends of Melvin. The shock of the young student's killing left him in a state of suspended reality. His own life had also been in danger and seeing how cheap life was to the gangsters he'd met, knew if Melvin got too irate a similar fate awaited him. Maybe even the killers wouldn't want him as a witness and pay a visit to silence him. Stephan was trying to come to terms with his existence, seriously questioning in which direction he should go.

He had spent the first night after the shooting on the office sofa in Producers Studio. He hadn't returned the key and knew the office was empty. He had lain awake most of the night with the shock of the events weighing on him. Jack and Reedo had picked up his car but Stephan was afraid to go back to Blem Gardens in case Melvin had learned where he lived. After a call with José, Stephan had been to the police the next afternoon for questioning, and it was a grim reminder of his predicament. Part of his sadness was from having had an inspiring talk with the young student and them both wanting to share more but having the chance brutally ended. The stark loneliness of his situation hurt so deeply that after seeing the police he called Lila and went over to her house.

Lila had welcomed him with a long, tight hug pressing every possible inch of her body against his. They ended up on her sofa curled up with their feet touching and after hearing his story Lila was visibly shocked at the near loss of her soul mate.

"This is so unbelievable. I always thought you were some kind of indestructible superhero, Wild West gunslinger kinda guy. I didn't know you were as good an actor as me." They both laughed.

"Sometimes you need to have a public face."

"I don't know what I'd do without you. You're so dear to me." Lila looked concerned.

"Nice to finally hear those words. I was starting to wonder if I had a place in your life."

"Of course." She paused a second to emphasize her words. "Yes, you do. I guess I was always afraid to show it. Thank god I didn't have to lose you to see how much I really care for you." She reached over and took both his hands in hers.

"I hope you know I've always thought of you as my perfect partner."

She smiled and leaned over to give a kiss and Stephan met

her halfway and it was intense and soulful, going on for an eternity. As soon as they came up for air they repositioned themselves, laying together. The many months of pent-up desire let loose in a sea of passion that relentlessly swept over them in waves of desire, drawing back only to wash forward again in another session of deep, caring lovemaking they both gave themselves to with abandon.

Stephan spent the night, and the next morning they were having a coffee in Lila's tree-shaded backyard, sitting in facing lawn chairs, with each other's feet in their laps.

"The shooter could have made an example out of me just as easy as that kid and I would have been seeing how much of my karmic debt was paid and how much was left to work out. Life is too short to be just a player, pretending to be cool," Stephan said.

"True. I've also been questioning my life lately, because this whole Hollywood dream machine game kills your soul if you play it too long, you know? Trying to look like a hot young thing, ready to put out at any occasion, isn't who I really am," Lila said with the last sentence sounding like a question with her Valley Girl accent.

"I know; you're really someone very special with such a potential on a whole other level. I bet once you get your teaching degree you'll able to turn so many people's lives around. Relax the body, relax the mind we used to say. Think how many people are so stressed from the scene here. You know, it's beaten you down long enough."

"You're right. This whole acting thing is fulfilling in some ways like learning how to identify with inner emotions and express yourself with confidence. Now I think I'm able to finally look beyond."

"Keep your eye on where you see yourself in five years and start to live the dream."

"Death is a powerful reminder of how little time we really have to accomplish anything of importance." Lila took a thoughtful sip from her coffee mug.

"So true. My friend Greasy Greg can play the cool guy role, always seeming to slide by without too many consequences like he can live forever. The only serious drawback is Greg's heroin addiction that he can't seem to shake, which is turning him into another person than the old friend who chased the truth with me."

"Why don't you try to visit Greg again? After what happened maybe you can seriously convince him to walk away from his dependencies once and for all."

"I've tried more than once with no results. Maybe I have to let Greg find his own way – I know he wants to. But you're right, at least one more visit wouldn't hurt."

"If he's such a good friend and sees how close you came to dying, he'll have the same reaction as me and understand how precious our short existence is."

"I think he already gets it. But I have to clear up some other stuff first. I already agreed with Miami Will to end our arrangement. He had no idea how out of control things had gotten and in no way wants to see me harmed. He's going to make the peace with Melvin so that'll be one less worry. Also, the police are aware of me, so an income based on illegal activities is not the most auspicious of occupations."

"What do the police know?"

"The two brothers at the shooting had to mention

there was another witness and when I was questioned by the homicide police in the Santa Monica courthouse building they told me not to leave town. In their eyes I'm just another guy on the scene who was partying with the cousins. What they want are the shooters. But the main issue of the moment is getting an alternative income. I have enough cash to live off of for a few months and with some concentrated effort I can probably pick up a job at a publisher or marketing agency."

"I'm here for you, however I can help," Lila said.

"Thanks for that." Stephan blew her a kiss and took one of her feet in both his hands, squeezing it. "Now I should get up to the office and get my papers and stuff before Malone clears it out."

Later on, as he was rummaging through the office looking at what he needed to take, Stephan was thinking how his life could also be simplified. With a stark picture of his existence, washed clean by his encounter with death, he could become like a monk and retreat to his humble home making it a writing sanctuary. He also wanted some time to let the emotions settle, to see the substance of his relationship with Lila and not jump into her arms out of a purely emotional dependency. He wanted to let their relationship mature slowly and richly in the true way he had imagined life with a perfect partner should be like. Now his writing would be enriched and once again having been touched to the core of his being, could convey some deep emotions to stir his readers with the feelings he wanted to share about the importance of finding peace inside.

The phone rang, breaking the reverie. Stephan was

surprised to hear James's voice.

"Hey, Stephan, what's up?" James said slurring his words.

"Wow – what a surprise." Stephan paused not sure what message he was going to hear. "It's been a long time."

"Yeah, too long. A lot of shit has gone down lately."

"You can say that again. Is everything okay? You sound pretty wasted." Stephan was concerned because he had never seen James out of control.

"Oh, man. I've been trying to drown my sorrows. I fucked up big time and Maria's run away. And I just heard from Frank that Greg's disappeared. I think they're together." The last words came out as an accusation.

"Are you crazy? She's totally in love with you. And besides, Greg's not that kind of guy," Stephan said with assurance.

"I don't know what to think anymore. I've been up for two days straight, loaded out of my mind."

"Hey, take it easy, man. What can I do to help?"

"Can you get up here today? You know Greg better than anyone and can probably figure out where he's hiding."

"Maybe." Stephan paused not sure how to tell James what happened. "Look, I was just part of some heavy shit and saw a murder go down—"

"What the fuck?" It was James's turn to be surprised.

"Listen, I'm okay but my head is also scrambled, so let me see how soon I can get away."

"Oh man, you're too good. Call me at the office when you sort your flight – and stay cool."

Stephan met James outside the arrivals area at the San Jose airport several hours later and they greeted each other with a hug.

"Oh man, it's good to see your face," James said. He was sobered up and while looking worn-out, his determined focus had surfaced again.

"It's been lightyears," Stephan said grinning.

"Let's catch up while we drive. I have a feeling something's wrong so there's not a lot of time." They walked quickly to the curb where James had his bus parked.

"Where do we start?" James asked once they were leaving the airport.

"We'll go over to Santa Cruz and check Greg's house for clues and ask around if anyone's seen him." The drive over the mountains to the coast allowed for the two friends to share their recent life experiences and put them into context. The conversation eventually came back to their time with the silent baba and the feeling of peace he had imparted.

James and Stephan drove by the harbor and found the small residential area where Maria's cousin Gloria lived. She was at home and let them know she had heard from Maria and that she was well but Maria hadn't disclosed where she was calling from. Even though she had been sworn to secrecy, after seeing the two friends' desperation, Gloria mentioned that Greg had helped Maria by offering her a place to stay. They felt better about the situation and tried his house, hearing from one of his new roommates they hadn't seen him for a couple of days. Next, they drove around downtown Santa Cruz hoping to spot someone who might have seen Greg.

"We've been over every square inch of this town and nobody's seen him in days. But I've got a feeling he isn't far," Stephan said after they had driven up and down every street in the center of town.

"At least Gloria confirmed Maria is getting help from Greg. Let's head over to Frank's. Maybe he's got some news."

They drove back over Highway 17 to the valley and went straight to Frank's house in the Cupertino foothills. They pulled in the parking area of the compound that was a combination of a large house, greenhouses and assorted outbuildings and parked the VW bus. Frank was under a car as usual and extracted himself. They stood in a circle talking as Frank wiped his hands on a greasy rag.

"Well, well – if it ain't the yogis from Muskogee," Frank said.

"Not so sure we're the saints you imagine," Stephan answered.

Frank replied, "After hearing about riots and James losing his lady maybe you're right."

James cut to the chase. "I need to find Greg because Maria's cousin said she's hiding with him at a house he has somewhere."

"Like I said when you called yesterday, I ain't seen the boy for weeks. The word on the street is that he's going down for the count," Frank said.

"What do you mean?" Stephan said.

"Kinda lost in an opium dream that always has a bad ending when it meets up with reality," Frank said. "Real sad."

"Holy shit, Maria could also be in danger," James said.

"Would any of the old crew know where his house is?" Stephan asked. "He told me once he bought some cabin in the middle of nowhere and it kinda sounded like it was in Marin or by Tahoe."

"I doubt anybody knows," Frank said. "Since he's been back he really went downhill. But come to think of it he did say he was working on a construction project and borrowed one of my pickups. That one over there." He pointed to a vintage vehicle painted vibrant green. "Some crazy ass scheme of making a dome out of old car hoods he read about in the *Whole Earth Catalog*."

They went across the courtyard to the ancient truck that had some scraps of wood and empty beer cans in the back. Stephan climbed in the cab and rummaged through the glove box without finding anything except a couple of old maps. He looked under the seat and retrieved a wadded-up receipt. He smoothed it out reading the print. "Hey, guys, check it out. A receipt from a Chevron station in Stinson Beach. It's dated May 10."

"That would be about the time he borrowed the truck," Frank said.

"Let's go check it out," James said.

"Good luck, amigos. Wish I could join you but my old man needs his ride ready in an hour," Frank said picking up his wrench and getting ready to crawl back under the car.

A couple of hours later James and Stephan were driving down a very rustic tree-lined stretch of Highway 1 in Marin County heading towards Stinson Beach.

"Can you believe it – it's been almost one year since we got back from India," James said.

"Seems like a lifetime. And here we are again on another quest," Stephan replied.

"What do you think the silent baba would tell us now?"

"Same stuff. Remember the oneness, everything is connected."

"Maybe Maria's leaving is to remind me again what's important. God, I feel like I've totally lost it. I don't know anymore if I should continue to pursue my dream or leave it for my love."

"I vote you keep them both. Maria would make a fine muse and keep you honest while you chase success."

"That's true. I'm sad she left but I'm not sure if it's because she ran off with Greg or because I really miss her."

"You love her, I can see that. Lighten up. She's probably using Greg to make you jealous so you'll pay attention."

"You're probably right. But all I want now is for her to be safe and happy." He paused and added, "Also Greg."

As they were driving down the Coast Highway they spotted the blue and red sign of a Chevron gas station coming up on the right.

"Check it out – the receipt I found was from a Chevron station," Stephan said.

They pulled in next to the gas pumps, got out and approached the clerk, a hippie chick in a small office who looked like Janis Joplin's little sister. She was wearing a low-cut floral print granny dress, a dozen strands of love beads and blue-tinted sunglasses with round lenses. James positioned himself by leaning on the desk. Stephan was more direct and stood in front of her where she sat on a low beat-up sofa with some underground newspapers scattered around on a neighboring cushion.

"Hi there," James said.

"Hellooo… how can I help you all?" the girl answered with a faraway voice.

"We're looking for a friend of ours named Greg. Maybe you've seen him – drives a silver Porsche with custom plates," James said.

"Oh yeah… Greasy – my favorite tantric massage partner." The answer came from dreamland and her eyes half closed with the sweet memory.

"Yes, that's him! Have you seen him lately?" Stephan asked.

"He stopped in here a few days ago. Had some chick with him who had long dark hair?" James sprang up from the desk he had been leaning against.

"Maria! Please, do you know where he lives – it's important we find him," James said.

"I never been to his place but he told me he's got a dome somewhere up in the hills where you can see the beach? Ya know?"

"Thanks, you've been a great help," James said and the two friends turned and ran back to the bus.

"Peace, brother!" the girl called after them.

James and Stephan had been driving up and down small country lanes for an hour and a half without any luck and were starting to feel their quest was futile when they drove past a dirt road with a padlocked chain across it. They slowed to see if there were any clues. About fifty yards along the dirt track was a two-way traffic sign of opposing arrows nailed to a tree.

"Hey! Check it out. Greg used to always draw two arrows on his hand to remind him of his breath going in and out when he smoked a joint. That must be it!" Stephan said.

James parked and they hiked up the dirt trail. A couple hundred yards along they came through the tree-lined tunnel and into a broad expanse of rolling hills with a simple wood cabin and a dome made out of various colored triangles of metal that could have been car hoods. Looking west over the countryside the dark blue ocean was visible in the distance, shimmering in the late afternoon sun. They looked around and inspecting the house saw some signs of recent occupancy with some leftover rice and vegetables in a casserole on the dining table. Moving to the dome, they circled it looking for the door. Further down the hillside they saw Maria facing the ocean, standing in front of an easel working on a painting. James ran over.

"Maria!" he called as he started across the hill.

Maria turned and looked like she wasn't surprised to see him and they embraced. She assumed that Greg had finally passed the word along where she was staying.

"Oh my love, it's so good to feel you again," she said gently.

"God, do you look good." He pulled back, studying her with an analytical gaze as if by examining her face he could see if she'd had an affair with Greg.

"What's the matter, something wrong?" Maria asked with a questioning look and tone of sadness.

James was searching for how to explain his doubts, not wishing to hurt her and break the special magic he felt rekindled. "It's Greg. I know he set you up here and—"

"Wait a second. I know what you're going to say. Greg and I are friends and that's it. If you had taken some time lately to talk with him you would know how we support each other," Maria said in a hurt tone.

"Oh, shit, I've fucked up again." He looked at her with teary eyes and hugged her once more. While he held her he was thinking about the test by fire he had witnessed in India and saw how in a split second he had made Maria prove her fidelity in the flames of his doubts. He kicked himself for rushing to judgment and realized how far he had strayed from the trust they had as a natural element of their relationship. He knew Maria's dedication to their being together was as unwavering as the faith of the young bride in India. James let out a sigh and stepped back holding onto Maria's hands.

James spoke slowly, not sure where to start. "Can you please forgive my stupidity? I must be the biggest fool on the planet not to see how precious you are."

"It's okay – we both needed some time to think. For me, it's clear we belong with each other." She tenderly brushed his tears away with her hands and then pulled him closer to look in his eyes, embracing him again in another tight hug.

"You're so right," James said into her shoulder where his face was buried.

"But what took you so long?" Maria asked slowly separating.

"What's going on? You don't seem surprised to see me."

"Didn't Greg tell you about our plan to hide me here?" Stephan joined them. "Hey there!"

"Hi Stephan – what a nice surprise." She quickly kissed him on the cheek.

"We haven't seen Greg. We played detective to track you down," James said.

"Oh my god. Something must have happened. After he dropped me off he was going to find you."

"Nobody's seen him for days," Stephan said. "We drove all over Santa Cruz and never found him and even Gloria doesn't know anything."

"He said he was going to clean himself up and get in touch with you," Maria said with a concerned tone.

"Let's get back to the valley and take it from there," James said.

They gathered up Maria's possessions and piled in the bus for the ride home. The three of them were wedged on the bench seat and the feeling between James and Maria was as if a veil had been lifted and a big step forward had happened. Maria couldn't keep her hands off James and talked a mile a minute about her days of being focused on her art and all the feelings it unlocked. She felt more grounded in her artist identity and knew she wanted to take it forward as far as she could. She explained that she was also able to see James for all his good and bad parts and really knew that they were meant to be life partners. When she said that, James tried to kiss her from where he was already tangled up in her embrace, almost going off the road in the process. Stephan shouted a playful warning and

James corrected his course. Maria turned away from James and gave Stephan a quick kiss on the cheek, telling him he also should trust in the universe to support his artistic side.

An hour and a half later they pulled into the drive of Maria's house and unloaded her baggage onto the lawn. She exchanged quick hugs with the two men and they got back in the bus and drove off. Maria's parents came out the front door to see what was going on and she ran up the walkway to embrace them.

24

THIS IS THE WAY THE WORLD ENDS

James came rushing into his living room where Stephan was sitting on the futon sofa with a phonebook and telephone calling everyone he could think of. "Frank got a call from a dealer in Santa Cruz an hour ago. The guy sold Greg some heroin which means he's still shooting up." He and Stephan both knew that after a detox a person's resistance is always lower and they exchanged worried glances.

"Let's go find him." James grabbed a set of keys off the dining table and headed for the garage where his old Mercedes was parked, with Stephan on his heels.

"Hey, man, what's this?" Stephan said looking at the car skeptically.

"It's a toy I bought. Don't worry, I've also had some professional driving lessons."

Stephan shook his head in amazement. "Let's rock and roll."

Half a minute later they were blasting along the on-ramp for Highway 17 as the car accelerated with a low growl, the motor only warming to its task. There wasn't a lot of traffic; rush hour hadn't peaked yet. When they crested the ramp and the incline leveled, the engine's power kicked in. They surged past the two slower lanes and with a quick shift flashed past any remaining cars. The Benz was swerving between trucks and cars as James wove the way through slow crawling traffic. He held to the legal sixty-five miles an hour until they whizzed past the gates of the old roadhouse on the edge of the Los Gatos city limits where the two large art deco cat statues watched dispassionately like sentinels.

Highway 17 was one of the most notorious roads for accidents in California. It wound through the Santa Cruz Mountains, home to trucks carrying two-ton loads of rock and gravel or monster lengths of massive redwood trees. Deep ravines lined with manzanita and poison oak waited hungrily on either side for fresh metal to consume. Combining this with tourists heading to the beach, commuters and every other type of local fool out for a cruise, made it a challenging task to get over the hill even in the best of conditions. James raced as fast as he could and, while not to the same extreme as the two racers had shown on their deadly contest, still made the miles fly by, shortening the time to get to the beach by half. Stephan was impressed at how well James controlled the car, expertly using its power and maneuverability. He couldn't help but think that somehow this race against the clock was karmic payback for what Greg had done to support James that fateful night with Tobias.

After scoring from the dealer in a run-down Victorian by the harbor Greg wanted a quiet place to fix up. His landlord had installed some guests in the extra bedroom of his house so Greg wanted to find another place he could crash, ideally undisturbed for a few days with no fear of being ripped off when he nodded off. Just wanted to enjoy a little taste of go-slow, country western, china white, scag, h-e-r-o-i-n.

He had done his latest round of self-rehabilitation with the resulting physical agony and mental torture triggered by the muscle spasms, chills, vomiting and diarrhea that were the easy part of the withdrawal compared to the bone-aching pain. Greg had wanted to keep his promise to Maria and make this last clean-up the one to get him going the right direction. When he returned to Santa Cruz he heard from Maria's cousin Gloria that James had been calling around looking for him, which was a first. Later, sitting in his beat-up house Greg tried to focus his thoughts and concluded with his still fuzzy thinking that the call could only mean that James was seriously angry with him for hiding Maria away, not an attempt at reconciliation. Distorted images of scenes he had witnessed where James could explode with little provocation floated in and out of his field of vision. Then a pang of guilt would flare up, jumbled in the other waves of emotion and Greg would think that he was probably deserving of a chewing-out having spaced out telling James where Maria was. The detox had taken longer than planned and the rustic cabin deep in the mountains above Big Sur was too nice to leave. His recently acquired way of dealing with issues and putting them into a manageable perspective with the assistance of a little dope could put him in the right frame of mind to hear James's remonstrations. It could also help to handle his living situation where a couple of strangers were sharing his house.

Greg forgot during his gradual return to mental clarity that after a episode of cleaning up a dependency, the body is returned to neutral and that starting a habit again at the same level where he left off was highly dangerous. The body could handle the original dosage of when he first started fixing but would once again need to build up tolerance to handle a stronger hit.

What Greg didn't know was that behind the invisible barrier he had been bumping against in his wheeling and dealing was the Italian Mafia and they considered Greg a pest. And because Tobias's father, Roberto, was affiliated with them for some peripheral dealings involving funny loads on his fishing boats, there wasn't much need for Roberto to offer too big a payoff to assure a low-level dealer supplied pure heroin when the opportunity presented itself. Set Greg up for a hot shot. Roberto had been getting updates on Greg as his eyes and ears were everywhere. The packet the dealer sold Greg that afternoon would have to be cut with a bag of lactose the size of a cement sack to make it average street purity of seven to eight percent, so even the tiniest dose would be deadly.

Greg blinked in the late afternoon daylight, unsure whether to head into town and cruise the Catalyst to find a friend or head for the broken-down hotels in the flats behind the amusement park roller coaster. The monkey wasn't entirely off his back and a little heroin would take the edge off. He moved in slow motion, like a zombie. By the time he reached the first motel he was sweating profusely, his shirt soaked through. He found a set of semi-permanent residents and had an argument with the junkies but the word on the street was that he was tainted goods that made them ask him to leave. At the second fleabag hotel, the occupants were either nodded out or gone in search of something to steal to pay for their habit, so nobody answered his pounding on the cheap door.

Greasy somehow found his way back downtown. He started a slow shuffle down the Pacific Garden Mall, past the Greyhound station, scanning for any familiar faces without any luck. The Mexican restaurant that had been a regular hangout was full with the happy hour crowd slamming margaritas with their chips and salsa. Greasy didn't feel optimistic and kept walking even though he knew one of the waiters was a shooter. Greg had once proudly showed Stephan while they were sitting at the bar, a worn spoon he fished out of the cutlery tray by the serving station that had a burnt backside from too much heating over a flame.

With the one-way traffic lurching stop and go along the Mall's narrow street, Greg paused to watch the old vibes player with freaky hair in front of the Cooper House shopping complex do his jazz show. He scanned the crowd for anybody he knew. As a longtime resident who knew everybody on the scene he spotted the perfect person to help – a doctor who had been a customer and owned a large house by the edge of the bay north of town where all the surfers went for the big waves. He approached the doctor sweaty and shaking and with his smooth-talking jive tried to find an opening to get an invite to the doctor's house. In the end he was practically begging as he had no other options and the doctor took pity on him and handed him a house key, also hoping for a little taste of go-slow when he got home later.

Stephan and James reached Santa Cruz and started patrolling the usual haunts, driving towards the roller coaster, heading for the hotels where Stephan had once cruised with Greasy. They knew that area would be Greg's first stop. At the second hotel, a loaded junkie only opened the door as far as the security chain would allow. In slowly molded words he said he had seen Greasy half an hour earlier. But they knew that junkie time was no time, so it could have been a week ago for all they knew. The pathetic creature had seemed fairly cognizant amidst his dream world visions, so they took his answer to be fairly accurate. They knew the next stop would be the Catalyst, so they crossed the river.

They parked along the one-way street dividing the Pacific Garden Mall and agreed to split up and meet back at the car in ten minutes. Stephan got lucky when he saw some people he knew from one of his visits sitting around an outdoor table drinking beer and listening to the afternoon jazz show. They had seen Greg twenty minutes earlier asking around for a place to crash for a couple of days. A quack doctor they all knew had given Greg the keys to his house and that was the last they saw of him. Stephan got the name and ran to a phone booth and looked up the address. Back at the car Stephan shared the update with James and they roared off.

It was slowly getting dark as they eased along the cliff

road with campers and surfer wagons lining the sides. They passed the statue of the noble Hawaiian who brought surfing to California where the inscription read: In memory of all surfers who have caught their last wave.

A minute later Stephan spotted the house number on a mailbox and visible down a short drive was a one-level ranch house set amongst a stand of scraggly cypress trees. They hastily pulled up in front and Stephan was out of the car first, pounding on the front door but with no answer. James ran around to the back with Stephan following. The kitchen door was locked but Stephan kicked it in with his boots. They ran through the house calling Greg's name and found him in the living room, laid back on the sofa with a syringe and other gear scattered on the coffee table.

Greasy was sitting at an angle with his head nodding forward. Stephan shook his shoulder and said, "Hey, man." Greg responded with a weak smile, raising his head slightly in recognition.

Greg spoke to them in a faraway dreamy voice. "What are you doing here? I thought you forgot about me. Your love is beautiful; I thank you for the gift." He paused, focusing his eyes. "You can call me Grateful Greg now." Then looking at James for a second with a slight smile, Greg quietly said, "Peace, brother. I'm cool, you cool?"

James placed his hand gently on Greg's shoulder and said, "Yeah, brother, I'm cool. Don't worry, we're going to take care of you."

Greg said softly, "Thanks, man," and then looked directly at Stephan. Greg's smile grew into the naughty grin that usually signaled a crude joke was coming. He winked and said, "Can you feel it?" He inhaled audibly like the two of them had taught students to connect with the movements of a yoga sequence and he looked Stephan in the eye. Then neutralizing his expression with his eyes taking a far-off look, Greg opened his mouth slightly and let out a rasping sigh, exaggerating the sound and gently pitched sideways on the sofa.

Stephan grabbed Greasy under the arms, pulling him upright saying, "Hey, man, don't leave us now. You can't go."

James swore. "Oh shit." He dashed over to a telephone on a side table and called 911 asking the operator for an ambulance because someone had overdosed. They picked Greg up, looping his arms over each of their shoulders as they walked him around the room trying to revive him. A couple of minutes later an ambulance arrived and one of the attendants immediately pulled an oxygen bottle out of the emergency kit and put it over Greg's face where he was laying again on the sofa.

"Sorry guys, he looks like a goner," the medic said with a sad tone.

Stephan answered through streaming tears, "No, he's not. He's just resting. He's going to be okay."

One of the other medics examining the packet of heroin dabbed the tip of his finger in the powder. He tasted it, quickly spitting on the floor and said, "Fuck me! It looks like your friend got a dose of uncut heroin. I'm going to give him a shot of something called Narcan to try and block the drug from shutting down his vital functions." The medic quickly pulled a hypodermic and small vial from his medical kit and gave Greg an injection.

"He's gonna make it. The guys got nine lives," James said.

The medic who had put the oxygen mask over Greg's face said as he felt for a pulse, "I think he's still breathing but we've got to get him to emergency, pronto, where we can give him a shot of adrenaline."

James consoled Stephan, putting a hand on his shoulder as they both kneeled on the floor looking at Greg lying peacefully on the sofa. "Hey, take it easy, he'll be alright."

"Yeah, I'm sure he will," Stephan sobbed.

Greg's left arm lay alongside him with his palm up. Stephan looked at the scars from where the tracks of injections had left their mark. The freshest point was still visible, with a drop of blood in the bend of his elbow. He pointed excitedly to just above Greg's wrist.

"Look at that." In fading ink there were two parallel arrows, pointing in opposite directions. Stephan remembered how when they first met, Greg would draw that image on his hand to remind him of the rhythm of his breath – the moment where the finite and infinite connected. Now it looked like he did the same for when he shot up.

"Greasy can be crazy at times but he always focused on peace and helping others," James said respectfully as he watched the attendants at work.

"Yeah, he ain't leaving us yet. There are a lot more people to help before he can finally check out to that great garage in the sky," Stephan said.

The two white-suited attendants gently lifted Greg onto a collapsible gurney and had a short consultation with the police officers who had just arrived before quickly getting Greg into the back of the ambulance. One of the attendants jumped in the back while the other dashed around the side to drive.

While the police examined the heroin the two friends walked outside to the edge of the trees and watched as the ambulance put on its flashing blue lights and sped off at a fast clip. Its plaintive, commanding wail got lost in the fog rolling in over the bluffs. The mist finally obscured everything, until it was just the two of them standing in a place with no time and no space.

25

IN TRUST WE'RE GOD

After they rescued Greg in Santa Cruz, James and Stephan had driven straight over to the hospital but they weren't allowed to see Greg because he was in intensive care. The doctors were able to keep him from slipping away and he had all his vital signs but hadn't regained consciousness. The doctors had warned that Greg could remain permanently in a coma or else simply wake up one day – there were no guarantees in life.

Stephan had visited every day after that, commuting from James's house where he was staying in one of the guest rooms. The vision of his friend hooked up to a drip feed and various monitoring devices saddened him. He took consolation in the fact that one day Greg could be back to his usual antics, without missing a beat. Greg's mother and sometimes Greg's father and brother supplemented his daily vigil. And occasionally Maria, her cousin, James or Frank would accompany Stephan, but Greg's condition remained unchanged. James would sit with Stephan reminiscing, or sitting quietly in meditation to see if perhaps their combined energies could draw Greg back to the waking reality, wanting to see Greg back jumping around.

The crew that filled James's Victorian house on the Sunday morning two weeks after Greg's overdose could have been a reunion of the brotherhood of forgotten yogis, called to the gathering by the flag waving on the pole out front – a large red Om symbol on a yellow background. The banner flapped in the breeze of a sunny day, framed by trails of high clouds, inviting all wandering sadhus and creative gypsies to a gathering of the faithful.

The day was intended to be light in tone, but there was still an air of melancholy as Greg's lively spirit was missing. He was the cosmic cheerleader who could rally up a group's flagging enthusiasm and reenergize it. He would provide a new direction, like a parent motivating a child by distracting it with another interest, to steer its attention away from where it was stuck. The event at James's house was a brunch that was meant to set a positive tone for moving on from the recent events and maintaining hope for Greg's eventual return. In true Greasy fashion, it resembled a party rather than a serious gathering.

Small groups formed around the house, with a couple of Greg's Santa Cruz friends including Emery hanging out in the backyard with Frank. They were sitting around a picnic table, eating macrobiotic and Italian snacks as an excuse to toss down some Chianti or beer. A mix of the engineering and programming teams revolved around Grok where he held court in the patio area. They were given to loud exclamations as they endlessly challenged each other, as conversations spiraled ever higher with each brainstormed concept a more advanced version than its predecessor. Greg's brother and parents were sitting at a patio table watching the crowd while a grill chef cooked burgers and hot dogs. James briefly watched the grill as occasional flames flared up, realizing he wasn't traumatized anymore from the fire in India.

Stephan was sitting with Lila on a bench by the Zen rock garden catching up. Lila leaned her head on his shoulder as they looked out over the field of small light brown stones raked into geometric patterns.

"I'm so happy you came up here. The longer we were apart, the more I felt we needed to be together," Stephan said as he stroked her hair.

"I guess we both need to let our brains shut down so the heart could open."

"You know I'm never going to let you out of my sight again?"

"Oh really? That won't be hard 'cause that's exactly the same plan I had in mind for you."

Stephan laughed and teased her a little. "But what about when you're filming the astronaut story? Just because you were able to get Eastwood to buy the script doesn't mean I can't visit you on the set."

"Well, you might just be hanging around supporting Maceo as a script consultant if you play your cards right."

"He did offer. I'm just happy to see him get the recognition he deserved."

"It wasn't easy with Sampson, was it?"

"Are you kidding? Development hell. But then seeing him on the news last week getting popped with enough coke to get all of LA county high and a house full of hookers seems like a fitting end to a Hollywood 'big concept' story."

Lila laughed. "Guess that and Maceo having had his script registered with the Writers Guild got him out of the scene pretty quick as well as his share of the studio advance."

The other pressing situation Stephan hoped to resolve had also had gone its natural course after the police managed to locate the two shooters. Harry had informed him that Malone had come under heavy fire from Hart, who on the inevitable discovery of the philandering, threatened to have all the legal muscle a millionaire mother could muster, come down on him like a ton of gold bricks. A divorce was quickly completed and Malone's house of cards came tumbling down which meant he was in survival mode with Stephan so far off the radar, their former partnership wasn't an issue any more. Also, Harry had told him the band was back gigging in cowboy saloons in the San Fernando Valley in yet another reincarnation, with the original singer and songwriter making demo tapes in a basement recording studio.

Stephan and James sat cross-legged on the futon sofa in the living room reviewing the past weeks' events with Lila and Maria who were seated on large cushions across the room from them. Lila had flown up that morning, with the two ladies hitting it off from the start. Over a long espresso-enhanced breakfast they shared their individual visions of art, both visual and dramatic with the similar challenges to the pure expression of a deep emotion. They bonded like sisters, spending an hour at the kitchen table discussing a tarot reading's symbols and other esoteric ideas before the hungry mob had descended. James lay back with his arms behind his head while Stephan sat upright, poised like a reporter with his journal open on a table in front of him.

After the wild ride and resulting reunion, there had been some time for reflection and looking at how to come together. James came to Stephan's rescue with an offer for Stephan to help out with the marketing communications for an electronic publishing software they were beginning to incorporate into the Eden machines, along with some new type of printers based on laser technology. Stephan would have to move back north but a regular job with a trusted friend sounded good. Stephan was getting back to his writing again and had gotten to the last part of the modified Ramayana story, where after all the battles and peace coming to the land his version of Rama was reunited with his wife. The adaptation was going well and with Lila at his side, he had fresh inspiration.

With the newfound attachment to his soul mate Lila, they decided after her role in the bicentennial story she would join Stephan in his move north. As a now fully certified Bilkem ShaktiFlow©®™ teacher, she could open her own corporate health service to cater for all the technology people staring at glowing cathode ray tubes all day, stressed from the constant barrage of deadlines and new releases all meant to be delivered the day before yesterday.

Maria shared an update. "In case any of you environmentally concerned individuals care, my father has not given up the fight to express his right to farm the land. He's now shifting the focus of his operations north. A cousin of his in Napa Valley was looking for a partner to expand his wine business with and they negotiated a deal.

Soon you will be seeing vintage Cappaletti Merlot and Rosé on the tables of all the finest restaurants in the land. If you're lucky, I may even invite you for a wine tasting." Maria laughed and went back to sketching quietly. Nobody mentioned Roberto but his fate was sealed. When word got around that he was complicit in Greg's death, Luigi had immediately cancelled any contracts with his trucking company and told the other farmers to do the same, essentially blackballing him from any contracts in the region.

James leaned forward to pick up his coffee and after taking a sip looked over at Maria. "Nice brew today." He paused while she gave him a look like saying excellence in coffee was normal. "You know, thinking about Greg I see life is about acceptance and recognizing every moment as being perfect, choosing to be happy about being alive. And if you can't appreciate the experience of life's goodness without it having to be taken away to remind you of how precious it is, then we all must be some serious hardcore morons." Maria smiled and nodded in agreement during the brief silence that followed.

"Speaking of the wheels of life turning as part of a perfect plan, we were going to go for a drive and leave you ladies in peace and quiet," Stephan said. "Frank is going to drive us over to the beach, a little more slowly this time, for a little cruise on the Coast Highway."

"You think that men are the ones who enjoy the pleasures of cruising? We ladies are going to follow along. My Fiat can match a Chevy any day of the week when it comes to mountain roads. It's not the car, it's the driver," Maria said proudly as Lila nodded in agreement.

"So how did you guess James wanted to go to San Gregorio beach and check out the nude sunbathers?" Stephan said.

"What!" Maria pretended to be shocked as she got up and made her way into the kitchen. "Anyone else want another espresso?"

"You think I can drink coffee and still be a yogi?" James asked Stephan with a smile, while raising his hand to signal Maria to include him.

Stephan laughed. "No concepts, man." He raised his coffee cup in a salute. "I don't want to shock you all but after everything that's happened, I'm going back to India before I start my new job. It's the most likely place to find that experience I'm after. I'm going to start by finding the silent baba again and see if he can point me to the source of his inspiration. He was onto to something real and maybe now I've evolved enough that he can explain things on a deeper level."

"Did you ask me if you could have the time off?" James joked.

"I think we should discuss putting the trip on your R & D budget," Stephan said. "And Lila said she will join me."

Lila jumped in. "That's right, I have some time before the astronaut film starts and after all my yoga classes, I thought I should go check out the source of it all."

"Please don't leave me behind," Maria said coming back from the kitchen holding a bag of coffee. "Lila told me earlier she was planning on going with Stephan, and I've been thinking about it. I also want to go along and see this amazing land and have some fresh inspiration."

"What, you want to go to India?" James said to Maria. "And what about me? You're all going to shove off and leave me alone?"

"You're the workaholic. Maybe it's time to get your priorities straight and regain your focus," Maria said playfully.

"Could be you're right. It's getting on Christmas – and with the holiday orders already in the works and mostly delivered I can leave Grok to watch the shop. I could catch up with you all in India over the holidays." He was met with a chorus of 'yeahs!'. "Why don't we rendezvous at the Blue Moon café in Dharamsala on New Year's Eve? We could start the year chanting some Om Mani Padme Hum's with the Tibetans, a few spins of those big prayer wheels and a good banging on some gongs to ring in the new and ring out the old. Would set us up well to track down the baba," James said.

Everyone agreed to the plan in an instant, laughing ecstatically and Stephan felt that old familiar tingle of infinite possibilities. The girls broke into an excited round of discussions on what they would wear, while Stephan opened his journal that was lying on the table to make a note. As he wrote, he watched the two opposing arrows drawn on his hand above the thumb as they danced up and down, once again reminding for that instant to be aware of his breath coming in and going out.

In a hospital room on the other side of the mountains not far from the coast, Greg lay in perfect stillness. An IV bag hanging from a metal stand occasionally gurgled and the soft hiss of the oxygen supply added to the ambient noise of the humming equipment. An attractive young nurse dressed in a crisp white uniform entered to look in on the patient and check the monitors. After assuring all the readings were stable, she paused and put one foot up on a visitor's chair. Knowing the patient was in a coma, she hiked her skirt up over the knee to adjust a stocking. The woman smiled at Greg's beatific expression as she smoothed out the silk material, thinking he'd be a cool guy to hang out with. The nurse left on her rounds and on the heart monitor that was showing a steady, almost flat line for the past ten days, a pointed peak momentarily appeared as Greg let out a gentle sigh.

Chris Corbett was born in the UK with the creative background of a grandfather who was a best-selling author in 1920s London as well as the first Artistic Director of the BBC and a great-grandfather who founded the Royal College of Music. Chris grew up in Northern California where he was educated at the University of California in Berkeley and in Santa Cruz. Moving to Los Angeles he worked for *Playboy Magazine*, Walt Disney and on an Academy Award winning film in addition to documentary film projects in Europe, America and India. He also owned a publishing business for eight years with a brother-in-law of one of the Beatles.

Since moving to Switzerland in 1986 he has been engaged in corporate communications at several multinational headquarters in Zurich. He has written articles and taken photographs for various print and on-line publications and had his fiction work published in a short story collection. Chris has also co-authored a best-selling non-fiction book: *The White Game – Achieving Peak Performance With the Power of Presence.*

He has been a student of yoga and meditation for many years, teaching his first yoga class in 1973.

ACKNOWLEDGEMENTS

I would like to thank some of the many people who helped make this dream a reality.

- Christopher Klim for providing early guidance and motivation to bring the book forward.
- John MacArthur, writing compatriot and word wizard par excellence for all his support, advice, and encouragement through the years, all the way to the finish line.
- Joseph Olshan whose writing wisdom and insightful editing shaped this tale into a real story.
- Helen Baggott for her perfect proofreading and insightful feedback.
- Henry Hyde who created a stylish and harmonious interior design that reflects the spirit of the book.
- The Jiva boys – Michael Lanning, Jack Reed, Tommy Hilton, Jim Strauss and Michael 'Reedo' Reed, for their many tales of life in a band on the run.
- Many thanks to Ian Graham and Günther Schöll for the gracious use of Kabir's Blues.
- Ram Dass for sharing with me his favorite parts of the Ramayana, providing inspiration and being here now. Maybe you're right and I really am a ten-headed demon!

- Professor Ron Geaves for his scholarly and experiential advice.
- Gary Girard who graciously allowed me to use his story *Attain This Knowledge* as the inspiration for the silent baba.
- Peter Schmidt who created some most awesome music for the song *One Out of Three*.
- Jeffrey Armstrong for his wise words inspired by the stars (in the sky) and encouragement.
- Stephen Stiteler for his friendship, support and healing energies to keep me tuned up.
- My son Philip, who always believed in this project and me – couldn't wish for a better son.
- My auntie Denise who never failed to give me encouragement and cracked the whip when I stalled.
- Anna Taylor from Taylormade for her creative excitement and showing me how every picture tells a story.
- The Guerdat brothers – Olivier, my attorney and Philippe my entertainment attorney, for their longtime support, feedback and passionate discussions.
- George Goen for providing his Hollywood narrative experience and Himalayan tour guide expertise.
- Those who offered me shelter to get on with the story telling: The Winslows in Southern California for the gracious use of their pool house (thanks sis!) and Javier Fernandez and family in Canos de Meca, Spain for putting me up in my favorite cabana.
- Greasy Greg – friend and fellow seeker – may you rest in peace.
- Prem Rawat for his continuous inspiration and support on my path to personal fulfillment.

The Merriest of Pranksters
Linda Ronstadt: "You're No Good"

Valley of the Heart's Delight
Bob Dylan: "It's Alright Ma"
Bob Dylan: "Subterranean Homesick Blues"
Günther Schöll: "Kabir's Blues"

Disco Inferno
Gloria Gaynor: "I Will Survive"
Hot Chocolate: "You Sexy Thing"
Silver Convention: "Fly Robin Fly"
Van McCoy: "The Hustle"

Welcome to L.A.
Creedence Clearwater Revival: "Proud Mary"
Lynyrd Skynyrd: "Sweet Home Alabama"

The Producers Studio
Frank Zappa: "Cosmik Debris"
The Doobie Brothers: "Takin' It to the Streets"
The Allman Brothers: "Midnight Rider"
Billie Holiday: "On the Sunny Side of the Street"
John Coltrane: "The Night Has a Thousand Eyes"

City of Angles
Peter Frampton: "Show Me the Way"
Elton John: "Don't Go Breaking My Heart"
America: "Horse With No Name"
The Rolling Stones: "Hot Stuff"
The Eagles: "Life in the Fast Lane"
Elton John: "Rocket Man"

Garden of Eden
Grateful Dead: "Truckin'"
The Beatles: "Back in the USSR"

Blem Gardens
Jiva: "World of Love"
The Allman Brothers Band: "Ramblin' Man"
Cher: "If I Could Turn Back Time"
Van Halen: "Dance the Night Away"
The Doors: "Light My Fire"
Joe Cocker: "Feelin' Alright"
Jiva: "Take My Love"
George Harrison: "Here Comes The Sun"
The Beatles: "Get Back"
Peter Schmidt: "One Out of Three"
Gary Wright: "Dream Weaver"

It's Only a Northern Song

The Rocky Horror Picture Show: "Time Warp"
Neil Young: "Down by the River"

Lila Mandeville and the Yogi of the Stars

Elvis Presley: "Suspicious Minds"
The Beatles: "Ballad of John and Yoko"

Money ist the Root of All Good

Bob Dylan: "Shelter from the Storm"
Led Zeppelin: "Stairway to Heaven"
Stevie Wonder: "As"

The Christmas Child

Herb Alpert: "A Taste of Honey"
Tom Petty and the Heartbreakers: "Breakdown"
Irene Cara: "What a Feeling"
The Eagles: "Hotel California"
Stevie Wonder: "Superstition"
The Who: "Baba O'Reilly"
Jiva: "Something's Going On Inside, L.A."
George Harrison: "My Sweet Lord"
Fleetwood Mac: "Go Your Own Way"

Baby Blue Flake Cosmic Colored Streamlined Baby

Dolly Parton: "Nine to Five"

Shifting Sands

Steely Dan: "Reelin' in the Years"
Bob Dylan: "Knockin' on Heaven's Door"
The Rolling Stones: "Brown Sugar"

Every Cloud Has a Golden Lining

Dr. John: "A Right Place at the Wrong Time"
Alice Cooper: "School's Out"
Ringo Starr: "It Don't Come Easy"
Led Zeppelin: "Good Times, Bad Times"
Crosby, Stills and Nash: "Long Time Gone"
George Harrison: "While My Guitar Gently Weeps"
Rod Stewart: "Do You Think I'm Sexy?"

If You Write It They Will Come

Fleetwood Mac: "You Make Loving Fun"
Stevie Nicks: "Nightbird"

Home Away From Home
Lynyrd Skynyrd: "Free Bird"

The Wrong Place at the Right Time
The Eagles: "New Kid in Town"

The Land That Time Forgot
Merle Haggard: "Okie from Muskogee"
Janis Joplin: "Me and Bobby McGee"

All Songs on Youtube

All Songs on Spotify

437